Should Vaccinations for Youth Be Mandatory?

Patricia D. Netzley

INCONTROVERSY

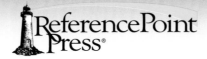
ReferencePoint
Press®

San Diego, CA

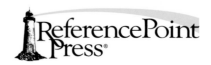

© 2013 ReferencePoint Press, Inc.
Printed in the United States

For more information, contact:
ReferencePoint Press, Inc.
PO Box 27779
San Diego, CA 92198
www. ReferencePointPress.com

LIBRARY OF CONGRESS CATALOGING-IN-PUBLICATION DATA

Netzley, Patricia D.
  Should vaccinations for youth be mandatory? / by Patricia D. Netzley.
    pages ; cm. -- (In controversy series)
  Audience: Grade 9 to 12.
  Includes bibliographical references and index.
  ISBN 978-1-60152-500-0 (hardback) -- ISBN 1-60152-500-1 (hardback)
  1. Vaccination of children--Popular works. 2. Vaccines--Popular works. I. Title.
  RJ240.N468   2013
  614.4'7083--dc23
                                                                   2012034789

Contents

Foreword

In 2008, as the US economy and economies worldwide were falling into the worst recession since the Great Depression, most Americans had difficulty comprehending the complexity, magnitude, and scope of what was happening. As is often the case with a complex, controversial issue such as this historic global economic recession, looking at the problem as a whole can be overwhelming and often does not lead to understanding. One way to better comprehend such a large issue or event is to break it into smaller parts. The intricacies of global economic recession may be difficult to understand, but one can gain insight by instead beginning with an individual contributing factor, such as the real estate market. When examined through a narrower lens, complex issues become clearer and easier to evaluate.

This is the idea behind ReferencePoint Press's *In Controversy* series. The series examines the complex, controversial issues of the day by breaking them into smaller pieces. Rather than looking at the stem cell research debate as a whole, a title would examine an important aspect of the debate such as *Is Stem Cell Research Necessary?* or *Is Embryonic Stem Cell Research Ethical?* By studying the central issues of the debate individually, researchers gain a more solid and focused understanding of the topic as a whole.

Each book in the series provides a clear, insightful discussion of the issues, integrating facts and a variety of contrasting opinions for a solid, balanced perspective. Personal accounts and direct quotes from academic and professional experts, advocacy groups, politicians, and others enhance the narrative. Sidebars add depth to the discussion by expanding on important ideas and events. For quick reference, a list of key facts concludes every chapter. Source notes, an annotated organizations list, bibliography, and index provide student researchers with additional tools for papers and class discussion.

The *In Controversy* series also challenges students to think critically about issues, to improve their problem-solving skills, and to sharpen their ability to form educated opinions. As President Barack Obama stated in a March 2009 speech, success in the twenty-first century will not be measurable merely by students' ability to "fill in a bubble on a test but whether they possess 21st century skills like problem-solving and critical thinking and entrepreneurship and creativity." Those who possess these skills will have a strong foundation for whatever lies ahead.

No one can know for certain what sort of world awaits today's students. What we can assume, however, is that those who are inquisitive about a wide range of issues; open-minded to divergent views; aware of bias and opinion; and able to reason, reflect, and reconsider will be best prepared for the future. As the international development organization Oxfam notes, "Today's young people will grow up to be the citizens of the future: but what that future holds for them is uncertain. We can be quite confident, however, that they will be faced with decisions about a wide range of issues on which people have differing, contradictory views. If they are to develop as global citizens all young people should have the opportunity to engage with these controversial issues."

In Controversy helps today's students better prepare for tomorrow. An understanding of the complex issues that drive our world and the ability to think critically about them are essential components of contributing, competing, and succeeding in the twenty-first century.

A Matter of Health?

In 2010 the United States had over twenty-seven thousand reported cases of pertussis, a contagious respiratory disease commonly known as whooping cough because it typically features a loud, wracking cough that can be strong enough to crack ribs. According to the Centers for Disease Control and Prevention (CDC), a federal agency that monitors diseases, this many cases in a single year had not appeared in the United States in decades. The number in California alone, over nine thousand, was the largest in the state since 1947.

Especially worrisome was that a significant portion of the victims were teens who had been vaccinated against whooping cough as children. This means they had been injected with the whooping cough vaccine—a preparation made using a component of the pertussis bacterium—so that their immune system would produce antibodies (disease-fighting blood proteins) against whooping cough. Stimulating the immune system in this way provides an immunity to disease, but the immunity can wear off. In the case of whooping cough, the vaccine's protection level drops by as much as 70 percent over five years. Therefore experts recommend that even after receiving a series of whooping cough shots as babies and toddlers, young people should receive a booster shot, or revaccination, at age eleven. Many of the teens affected by the 2010 epidemic had not gotten this shot.

Once California officials realized the cause of the whooping cough outbreak, they passed a law requiring students in grades seven through twelve in a public or private school to show proof that they had received the booster shot. Students who did not have the required proof would not be allowed to attend school. In this way, California was acknowledging the fact that many people fail to get a vaccination unless it is mandatory—that is, required by law—in order for them to get something they want, such as school admission or a particular job. As an example of this, the CDC reports that as of 2010 only 8 percent of adults had gotten a whooping cough booster shot, which is strongly recommended but not mandatory.

Serious Consequences

Many adults who do not get recommended vaccinations and booster shots fail to understand how serious some contagious diseases can be. Whooping cough, for example, can cause pneumonia, which is often deadly in infants that have not yet been vaccinated. Veronica and Sean McNally of Michigan, for example, never imagined that the fact that neither had received a whooping cough booster shot as adults would lead to the death of their baby, Francesca. In 2012 Veronica contracted whooping cough, then passed it on to her infant daughter, who was not yet old enough to be fully immunized. Soon the baby's lungs were so compromised that doctors had to put her on a respirator, but the child still died.

Afterward the McNallys created the Franny Strong Foundation, named for their daughter, to promote the message that everyone should be vaccinated against whooping cough because the disease can kill young children. "I had a child, and my child would be here but for this tragic and terrible disease," Veronica McNally says. "This foundation is really, for the rest of my life, my tribute to her life and to what happened to her."[1]

Teens and adults rarely die from whooping cough, but they can still suffer because of the disease and spread it to others. For example, journalist Paula Simons, who contracted the disease in her early twenties, says, "I have never in my life been so sick. The cough would abate during the day—but in the night, and in the early morning, it was unbelievable. I couldn't get my breath. I felt like I was drowning. Sometimes, I coughed so hard, I vomited. My rib cage felt as though it were being pulled apart. Still, I was young and stupid. I dragged

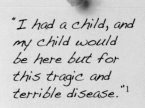

"I had a child, and my child would be here but for this tragic and terrible disease."[1]

— Parent Veronica McNally, who lost an infant to a whooping cough infection.

myself to work every day, foolishly spreading bacteria as I went."[2] Like a lot of other people, Simons had no objection to getting vaccinated, she just did not realize her protection had worn off and that she needed a booster shot.

Anti-vaccination Sentiments

Some individuals, however, do not believe that vaccinations are necessary, or they believe that childhood vaccinations can be delayed until later. According to a study reported by the American Academy of Pediatrics in November 2011, 13 percent of parents do not support the vaccination schedule recommended by the CDC and most doctors. Of these, 17 percent think that neither they nor their children should ever be vaccinated with any vaccine, while 53 percent think that while a few vaccines are necessary most are not. And even among parents who do follow the recommended vaccination schedule, 22 percent are not sure that doing so is safe for their children, and 28 percent would support delaying vaccination until children are older.

Proponents of vaccination say that such beliefs are often the result of fear and distrust of the medical establishment, but these feelings are nothing new when it comes to vaccinations. When physician Edward Jenner developed the first vaccine in England in the 1790s, people reacted in much the same way—in no small part because of how the vaccine was administered. Jenner's vaccine targeted smallpox, a highly contagious and frequently fatal disease caused by the variola virus. Its symptoms include the eruption of painful pus-filled blisters, and the process by which Jenner vaccinated children—a process called variolation—seemed bizarre and somewhat frightening. He took fluid from beneath cowpox blisters, which he had discovered would provide immunity to smallpox in humans. He then made a small cut in the skin of the child's arm and inserted the fluid under the skin.

By the time the vaccine was developed, smallpox had killed at least 500 million people throughout the world. Therefore many public officials supported Jenner's work and quickly established smallpox vaccination programs not only in England but in other countries as well. As a result, within twenty years of the develop-

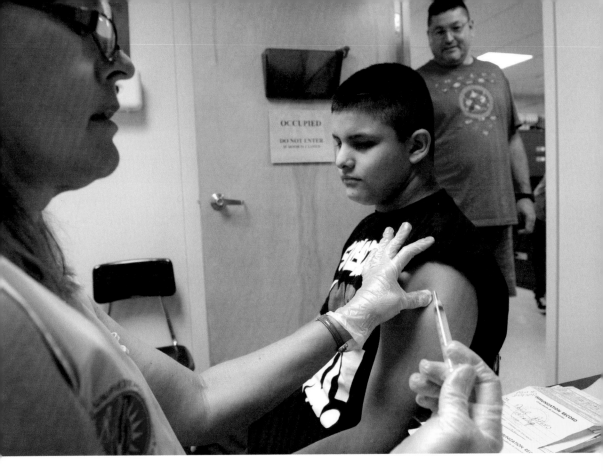

ment of variolation, deaths from smallpox were cut in half.

Nonetheless, in many countries religious leaders opposed vaccination efforts in the belief that the disease had been sent by God to punish sin and that anyone who sought to prevent these punishments was in league with the devil. Some religious leaders also said the vaccine was "unchristian" because it involved putting part of an animal (the blister fluid of a cow) into a human. At public rallies, those opposed to vaccines—today called anti-vaccinationists, anti-vaxxers, or vaccine refusers—also stoked fears among the populace that vaccines were dangerous.

Public officials responded to these fears by establishing mandatory vaccination laws; the first such law was enacted in England in 1853. Initially this law required infants up to three months old to get a smallpox vaccination, but in 1867 the government extended the age requirement to fourteen years and mandated a fine for parents who failed to comply with the law. Parents who could

A Southern California student receives his whooping cough immunization before the start of a new school year. Many school districts now require proof of immunizations in hopes of preventing outbreaks such as the whooping cough outbreak that spread through California in 2010.

not afford to pay would see their possessions sold at public auctions, and if the proceeds still did not pay off the fine, the parents would be jailed.

Public Protests

In response to this mandate, an anti-vaccination movement developed in England and gained supporters as the years passed. For example, at an anti-vaccination demonstration in 1885, roughly eighty thousand to one hundred thousand people marched in protest against vaccinations. As a result of such efforts, England eliminated the penalties for failing to vaccinate and allowed parents who objected to the vaccine for religious or personal reasons to avoid getting their children vaccinated.

In the United States, resistance to a smallpox vaccination program began even before the first mandatory vaccination law was enacted in Massachusetts in 1809. By that time, an anti-vaccination society in Boston, Massachusetts had been speaking out against Jenner's work for eleven years, even arguing that doctors performing vaccinations should be tried for attempted murder. Others launched legal challenges to mandates as they occurred, but in 1905 the US Supreme Court decided that states had a constitutional right to pass vaccination laws.

In other places, resistance to mandatory vaccination was expressed through violence. In 1904 in Rio de Janeiro, Brazil, the Vaccine Revolt occurred in response to a new vaccination law that allowed health workers, accompanied by police, to go into people's homes to forcibly inject them with smallpox vaccine. During the subsequent riots, at least 110 people were wounded and 30 were killed before officials got things back under control—after which the forced vaccination program resumed, and smallpox was eventually eradicated from the city.

Opposition and Consequences

Because vaccination programs are typically successful at lowering disease rates, many governments have established such programs despite public resistance. In the United States, for example, all fifty states and the District of Columbia have mandated vaccination programs, though the diseases being targeted vary from state to state. However, every state recognizes that some people have an immune system that cannot tolerate a vaccine, and these individuals are exempt from vaccination. Many states also provide exemptions for people who oppose vaccination on the basis of their religious beliefs, and a few states provide exemptions for philosophical or personal beliefs as well.

Anti-vaccinationists applaud these exemptions, but they believe that *all* people should be allowed to reject vaccinations if they so choose. They point out that vaccines are not 100 percent safe because some people experience serious side effects after being injected, and they argue that mandates are a threat to freedom. For example, Barbara Loe Fisher, a leader of the US anti-vaccination movement, says: "If the State can tag, track down and force individuals against their will to be injected with biological products of unknown toxicity today, then there will be no limit on which individual freedoms the State can take away in the name of the greater good tomorrow."[3] But a failure to vaccinate can have grave consequences. Studies have shown that children whose parents refused to get them vaccinated for whooping cough, for example, were anywhere from eight to twenty-three times more likely to contract the disease. This can put others in the population at risk. In 2012, for example, more than 50 percent of all whooping cough cases came from six states (Pennsylvania, Wisconsin, Washington, Texas, Arizona, and Ohio) that offer a personal or philosophical exemption from vaccinations. Some of these cases resulted in infant deaths.

"If the State can tag, track down and force individuals against their will to be injected with biological products of unknown toxicity today, then there will be no limit on which individual freedoms the State can take away in the name of the greater good tomorrow."[3]

— Prominent anti-vaccinationist Barbara Loe Fisher.

The controversy over mandatory vaccinations essentially comes down to a debate between those who believe that individual rights outweigh public need and those who say that in matters of health, the public good takes priority over individual choice. With such strongly held views on both sides, the debate is likely to continue.

Facts

- An epidemiologist is a person who studies the spread of disease.

- Epidemiologists use the word "cluster" to refer to a group of disease cases that occur during the same period in the same area and that seem greater in number than one would expect to see.

What Are the Origins of the Modern Vaccination Controversy?

In 1979 the World Health Organization (WHO) announced a public health milestone: the eradication of smallpox. The last known naturally occurring case of smallpox was identified in Somalia in 1977. No naturally transmitted cases of smallpox have occurred anywhere in the world since that time. The WHO attributes this achievement primarily to global immunization efforts.

Other diseases, though not classified as eradicated, have been largely eliminated or are considered under control either worldwide or in specific regions thanks to immunization programs. These include rubella, measles, and polio. For example, rubella—a viral disease that causes flu-like symptoms and a rash—is thought to have been eliminated in North and South America. (WHO experts are currently working to verify that rubella has not appeared in the Americas since 2009.) Many countries have targeted rubella in their vaccination programs because infection during pregnancy can lead to miscarriage, stillbirth, or birth defects.

The Swine Flu Scare

These successes have not allayed the fears of those who believe that vaccines do more harm than good. The current level of distrust of vaccines began in large part in the United States because of a 1976 government response to the threat of a swine flu epidemic. Swine flu is a respiratory virus that comes in several varieties, or strains. One of these strains was involved in a 1918 pandemic—an epidemic affecting several countries—that killed at least 50 million people worldwide. So when a soldier at the Fort Dix army base in New Jersey died of a similar strain of flu in February 1976, federal officials were concerned that another flu pandemic was on the way. In the hope of preventing such a pandemic, President Gerald Ford mandated the inoculation of everyone in the United States against the flu—roughly 220 million people—as part of a $135 million vaccination program.

The flu vaccine was then rushed into production, with manufacturers skipping the usual rigorous and time-consuming testing so that the program could begin as soon as possible. Meanwhile, Congress agreed to protect manufacturers from lawsuits if their vaccine hurt anyone. Unfortunately, this is exactly what happened when the program launched in October 1976. Within days of lining up at health clinics, schools, and firehouses to get a flu shot, some of those vaccinated reported disturbing symptoms that included respiratory distress and muscle weakness. A few elderly people suffered heart attacks and died right after getting their shot. Health experts soon realized that the vaccinations were somehow causing Guillain-Barré syndrome (GBS), a rare but potentially fatal neurological illness whereby the body's immune system mistakenly attacks part of the nervous system. (Poorly understood, this syndrome can also develop after a surgery or serious infection.)

In commenting about the event in hindsight, David J. Sencer, who was the director of the CDC in 1976, says, "If we had [more] knowledge then, we might have done things differently. We did not know what sort of virus we were dealing with in those days. No one knew we would have Guillain-Barré syndrome. The flu vaccine [for other influenza infections] had been used for many years without that happening."[4]

Extreme Enforcement

In 1909 New York health officials helped establish just how far the government can go in protecting the public from contagious diseases. That year, six people in a family spending the summer in Oyster Point, Long Island, contracted typhoid fever, a potentially fatal disease caused by a bacterium that can be spread through food contaminated by an infected person. Investigators soon determined that the family's temporary cook, Mary Mallon—even though she herself did not seem sick—was the source of their typhoid and that of others she had worked for in previous years. The first American identified as a healthy carrier of typhoid, "Typhoid Mary" was ordered never to work as a cook again. When she violated this order, officials imprisoned her for the rest of her life on North Brother Island in New York's East River, where a hospital had been established in the 1850s to quarantine smallpox victims.

But because of the GBS cases—initially around fifty were reported in several states—the government ended the mandatory vaccination program on December 16. By then, over 40 million people had received a swine flu shot. Over five hundred of them ultimately developed GBS, and twenty-five died of GBS-related complications. Because the vaccine's manufacturers had no liability for these damages, the US government took responsibility for them, paying out nearly $100 million to victims or their survivors.

Successful Programs

This disaster, along with the fact that the predicted pandemic never materialized, made many people suspicious of government warnings regarding health issues. Proponents of vaccination say this is especially unfortunate because prior to the 1976 flu scare most Americans had positive feelings about vaccination programs. During World War I, for example, the number of soldiers killed by influenza (forty-four thousand) was almost as high as the number lost in battle (fifty-five thousand). By the time of World War II, however, a mandatory influenza vaccination program largely prevented the spread of the disease among the troops.

As a result, when these soldiers returned home they supported postwar inoculation efforts. They especially welcomed widespread trials of vaccines against polio, a crippling and sometimes deadly disease that struck at least 20,000 children in the United States every year. Developed in 1952 during a polio outbreak that afflicted 58,000 (and another 35,000 the following year), these vaccines—one injected, one given orally via a sugar cube—were administered to over a million schoolchildren in 1954, and the results were so successful that in 1955 the US began launching mass immunization campaigns against polio. As a result, in 1957 the number of US cases of the disease dropped to 5,600, and by 1964 there were only 121 cases. Retired pediatrician Bob Guinter of Collierville, Tennessee, recalls the reaction to the vaccine that could prevent polio: "I am old enough to remember a grade-school classmate who needed leg braces because of weakness caused by polio. And I can still remember the look of almost religious zeal on my mother's face as she took us to get our sugar cube containing precious drops of polio vaccine." He adds that he has never seen a case of polio among any of his patients in more than thirty-four years as a doctor. "Immunizations have worked so well that many young parents today have never known a family whose child had a vaccine-preventable illness,"[5] Guinter says.

Despite these successes, the swine flu scare led some people to start shunning vaccinations. For example, when the government called on people to get a flu vaccination in 2009 because of a possible epidemic, Warren D. Ward, who was in high school in California during the 1976 scare, said, "I'm not getting it. I felt back then [in 1976] like it was a bunch of baloney."[6]

"Immunizations have worked so well that many young parents today have never known a family whose child had a vaccine-preventable illness."[5]

— Retired pediatrician Bob Guinter.

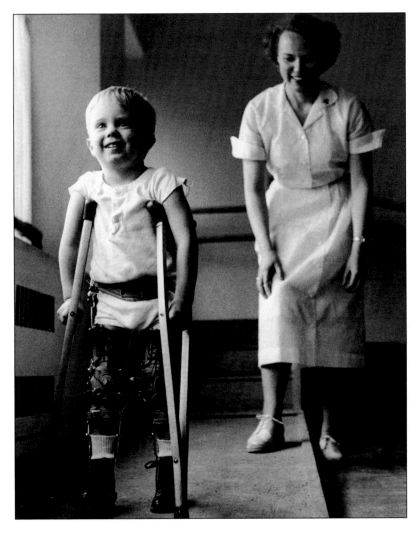

A boy who contracted polio, a crippling and sometimes deadly disease, practices walking with crutches and leg braces in the 1950s. A mass vaccination effort that began in the 1950s dramatically reduced polio cases in the United States.

School Attendance

Mandates were created to combat such sentiments, at least regarding contagious diseases known to put people's lives at risk. All states and the District of Columbia have at least some mandated vaccinations, and all of these mandates are tied to school attendance. For example, California law mandates that students be vaccinated for diphtheria, hepatitis, influenza, measles, mumps, pertussis, polio, rubella, and tetanus. Students who cannot provide proof of vaccination are not allowed to attend classes. Parents have challenged such laws, but so far the US Supreme Court has upheld them.

However, all states and the District of Columbia also acknowledge valid reasons for not mandating certain vaccinations for certain children. In fact, all states allow a person whose immune system is weak to skip all vaccinations, and anyone with a proven allergy to a particular vaccine is not required to be injected with that vaccine. All states except Mississippi and West Virginia also allow people to refuse vaccinations if getting vaccinated runs counter to their religious beliefs, and twenty-one states currently allow exemptions based on philosophical or personal beliefs.

Combination Vaccines

The number of states allowing philosophical exemptions has risen in recent years because of controversies related to combination vaccines, which are vaccines that inoculate someone against more than one disease in one shot. The advantage to using a combination vaccine is that a young person needs fewer shots in order to be fully immunized, which means fewer painful injections and fewer visits to the doctor. However, a small but growing number of health professionals believe that combination vaccines might be too hard on the immune system, especially in infants.

This belief arose largely because of suspected problems with the DPT vaccine, which protects against diphtheria, pertussis, and tetanus. The diphtheria vaccine was first marketed in the 1920s, pertussis in 1906, and tetanus in 1933, but these individual shots were largely set aside after the DPT vaccine became available in 1946. Problems surfaced almost immediately. In 1948 a study carried out by researchers at the Harvard Medical School and conducted at Children's Hospital in Boston found that some of the children who received the DPT shot developed severe neurological problems. These results were published in the journal *Pediatrics*, but the vaccine remained on the market, and the federal government continued to recommend the vaccine as the best way to vaccinate infants.

In the 1970s, however, several well-publicized reports of children suffering convulsions, brain swelling, and brain damage after

"The DPT vaccine had one of the worst failure rates of any product submitted to the [FDA's] Division of Biologics for testing."[7]

— Charles Manclark, a scientist with the FDA.

a DPT injection led to a surge in anti-DPT sentiments among parents. This occurred not only in the United States but also in Great Britain, Sweden, and Japan, the latter of which had several cases of infant death that appeared to be related to the vaccine. In response, Japanese and US researchers launched an effort to create a new version of DPT.

Abandoning DPT

By this time, officials with the National Institutes of Health (NIH) and the Food and Drug Administration (FDA) had admitted that the DPT shot had major issues. In 1976, for example, Charles Manclark of the FDA stated that "the DPT vaccine had one of the worst failure rates of any product submitted to the [FDA's] Division of Biologics for testing."[7] Studies had also determined that the problem with DPT was in the pertussis portion—or more specifically, in the way the whooping cough portion of the vaccine was created.

Vaccines can be made in several ways, as long as the resulting immunization stimulates the body to produce antibodies to the disease. In the case of the DPT vaccine, whole cells of the pertussis bacteria were used to produce the immune response, but they triggered a reaction so extreme that it could damage the brain. The Japanese researchers found that if purified cell components were used instead of whole cells, these side effects could be avoided.

As a result, Japan abandoned the DPT vaccine in favor of DTaP (diphtheria, tetanus, and acellular, or cell-free, pertussis) for babies in 1981, and some other countries did the same. However, it was not until 1997 that babies in the United States received DTaP instead of DPT. Some people believe that this delay was based on monetary concerns. For example, in a 1996 editorial commenting on the CDC's recent approval of the DTaP vaccine's use for infants, Harold Stearley, a nurse, wrote:

A purified vaccine [DTaP] is available that's virtually reaction-free, and has been produced and used in other countries for over 15 years, using technology the U.S. abandoned in the 1970's. The catch: it costs $9 more per injection. While most parents would happily cough up the additional nine bucks to ensure their children's safety, drug companies have lobbied to delay the use of the purified vaccine (acellular) for as long as possible—it might cut into their inflated 50 percent profit margins per vaccination.[8]

Others point out that at the time, the United States continued to use DPT because studies did not provide conclusive evidence that the vaccine caused harm. In fact, some say there is still no such evidence. Nonetheless, publicity over cases where children suffered serious health problems right after receiving their DPT vaccinations fueled controversy over which was more dangerous, the whooping cough disease or the vaccine, and the government was eventually forced to address parents' concerns.

Parental Activism

One example of a well-publicized case involving the vaccine was that of four-month-old Julie Schwartz of Chevy Chase, Maryland, who received her third DPT shot in July 1981. Later that day, she had a severe seizure, and when her parents took her to the emergency room, doctors there blamed the seizure on the inoculation. Over the next two years Julie suffered roughly fifty additional severe seizures and several minor ones, and at eleven months old she lost all movement on her right side, probably as the result of a stroke. With physical therapy she regained some abilities, but shortly before her third birthday she had a seizure and a heart attack and died.

In the hope of preventing other such tragic deaths, Julie's parents, Jeff and Donna Schwartz, formed a group called Dissatisfied Parents Together (DPT). While promoting the group in 1985, Jeff Schwartz said, "I am not trying to avenge [Julie's] death by going on a vendetta against the drug companies and forcing them to cease manufacturing vaccines that help rid the world of childhood diseases."[9] Instead, the goal of this group and others was to make parents aware that if a child reacted

"I am not trying to avenge [Julie's] death by going on a vendetta against the drug companies and forcing them to cease manufacturing vaccines that help rid the world of childhood diseases."[9]

— Jeff Schwartz, cofounder of Dissatisfied Parents Together.

to the first of the three DPT vaccination shots with convulsions, collapse, or high-pitched screaming, the child should receive no more shots.

Because of such awareness campaigns, the US Senate held a hearing in 1985 on DPT vaccinations, and federal health officials admitted that roughly thirty-five thousand children a year had suffered neurological damage as a result of the vaccine. Others dispute this, some arguing that unidentified health problems and/or vaccinating a child too early were to blame for the injuries rather than the DPT vaccine.

No Liability

In the 1980s a few hundred parents who believed their children had been harmed by the vaccines sued vaccine manufacturers for damages. One such lawsuit concerned a three-month-old who had become paralyzed from the waist down after receiving a DPT shot. Even though no other cases of this kind of paralysis had been associated with DPT, the jury awarded the child's parents $1.13 million.

Such judgments led many pharmaceutical companies to stop making vaccines. Between the 1970s and 2004, the number of US vaccine manufacturers dropped from twenty-five to five, and by 1985 only one US manufacturer was offering the DPT vaccine. By this point, federal officials had become concerned that eventually no private company would want to supply US physicians with vaccines. Consequently Congress passed the National Childhood Injury Act of 1986 to protect companies from lawsuits related to federally approved vaccines. Upheld by a US Supreme Court ruling in February 2011, the law also created a federal program, the National Vaccine Injury Compensation Program (NVICP), to compensate victims of side effects linked to childhood vaccinations. This program caps damages, which means that a victim can get no more than a certain amount for a certain type of claim, and the payouts are financed by a tax on every vaccine dose.

The Wakefield Incident

Once pharmaceutical companies were absolved of vaccine-related liability, a public already concerned about vaccine safety became

Contaminated Polio Vaccine

Certain batches of polio vaccine produced prior to 1963 were contaminated with simian virus 40, or SV40, a virus found in both monkeys and humans. In most monkeys it causes no symptoms of disease. However, when hamsters are injected with the virus they develop cancerous tumors. Consequently, after the virus was discovered in 1960 in rhesus monkey kidney cells used to make polio vaccines, US officials suspected that 10 to 30 million Americans might have been exposed to the virus. However, since then experts have disagreed on whether SV40 does cause cancer in humans.

Long-term studies of those who were vaccinated with contaminated vaccine indicate that they are at no greater risk of getting cancer than anyone else. In one such study in Germany, 886,000 people who received the contaminated vaccines as infants were followed for twenty-two years. Another followed 10 percent of the exposed population in the United States for thirty years. However, a significant percent of certain rare tumors found within people exposed to the contaminated vaccine have shown traces of the SV40 virus within them, and the National Cancer Institute is continuing to investigate this situation.

even more distrustful of vaccine mandates. Into this climate of distrust came a research paper that ignited anti-vaccination passions. Published in 1998 in the respected medical journal the *Lancet*, the paper suggested that the combination vaccine against measles, mumps, and rubella (MMR) might be triggering a bowel problem that in turn might be causing the onset of autism. Autism is a developmental disorder characterized by behavioral problems related to social interaction.

The main author of the paper was gastroenterologist Andrew Wakefield of the United Kingdom (UK). Wakefield theorized that the MMR shot overloads the immune system, weakening it to the point where the measles virus can attack the intestines and cause them to shed proteins that can damage the brain. Wakefield argued for vaccinating against each disease individually until more research could be conducted.

The media immediately seized upon the suggestion that MMR shots might be causing autism, and many parents who heard the news refused to take their children for MMR vaccinations. Meanwhile, many in the medical profession attacked Wakefield's work. Articles critical of Wakefield attacked not only his conclusions but the fact that his study only involved twelve children, which many experts believe is not enough for research of this nature.

Among Wakefield's toughest critics was British journalist Brian Deer, who for years after the publication of Wakefield's *Lancet*

Andrew Wakefield's 1998 journal article linking the measles-mumps-rubella vaccine (MMR) to autism fueled a nascent anti-vaccination movement. In 2010 a panel of medical experts found Wakefield (pictured) guilty of ethical violations, including falsifying data, in his vaccine research.

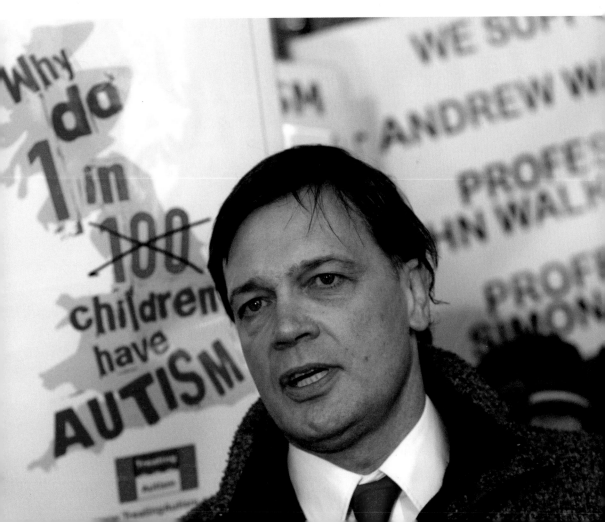

article fought to have the work repudiated. Deer accused Wakefield of unethical behavior, such as neglecting to mention signs that the subjects of his study were already developing autism prior to getting their MMR vaccinations. For example, one mother reported that her child had imperfect hearing, a possible indication of autism since children with autism have problems listening to people. However, Wakefield says he did not mention this because the child had an ear infection, which Wakefield believes was the reason for the diminished hearing.

Wakefield similarly disputes other accusations leveled by Deer and others. In 2010, after a nearly three-year study initiated largely because of Deer's efforts, a panel of medical experts found Wakefield guilty of ethical violations, including falsifying data. As a result, Wakefield lost his right to practice medicine in the UK. That same year, the *Lancet* retracted Wakefield's original article, and in 2011 the *British Medical Journal* published a series of articles by Brian Deer defending the decision.

Lasting Distrust

But parents whose children developed autism shortly after their MMR vaccinations still believe Wakefield is right. He also has some supporters in the medical community, especially among those who deal with the gastrointestinal problems of children with autism. For example, Judy Converse, a nutrition specialist who has worked with autistic children for years, complains that many of those criticizing Wakefield have not even read his original study or others supporting his work. She says, "I challenge physicians out there to pause, breathe, read the studies, and wonder. Think it through: What if he's right?"[10] Converse suggests that Wakefield has been the target of criticism because the pharmaceutical industry cannot allow people to think its combination vaccines might be harmful.

Wakefield's supporters have also noted that Brian Deer was attacking Wakefield while working for wealthy media mogul Rupert Murdoch, who has financial ties to the pharmaceutical industry. Therefore some of these supporters, including health

"We can only imagine what has been going on behind closed doors in the world of pharmaceuticals."[11]

— Health expert and nutritionist Catherine J. Frompovich.

expert and nutritionist Catherine J. Frompovich, have called for an examination into what role Murdoch's business empire might have played in Wakefield's downfall. Suggestions of impropriety have been magnified by recent government investigations into bribery and corruption involving Murdoch's company. Given these accusations, Frompovich says, "We can only imagine what has been going on behind closed doors in the world of pharmaceuticals."[11]

Frompovich has no evidence to support her suspicions, however, and on his website Deer explains that his motivation for going after Wakefield was a personal mission to end a "global crisis" caused by parents refusing to vaccinate their children. He adds, "I was glad to expose him as dishonest and a research cheat, preying on vulnerable families."[12] But the fact that Frompovich and others have suspicions about Deer is indicative of the level of distrust that currently exists in regard to vaccines and their makers.

Facts

- A hundred years ago young children received only one vaccine—against smallpox; today the CDC says that during the years between birth and age six, children should receive twenty-seven shots intended to fight thirteen diseases, as well as a yearly influenza shot.

- The diseases currently targeted by the CDC's childhood vaccination recommendations are chicken pox, diphtheria, Hib, hepatitis A, hepatitis B, influenza, measles, mumps, pertussis, polio, pneumococcus, rotavirus, rubella, and tetanus.

- Before the measles vaccine was developed in the mid-1950s, almost all children in the United States contracted the disease by the age of fifteen.

- Vaccine batches have lot numbers so that if the CDC determines that a particular batch is less effective than others it can be recalled from physicians' offices, clinics, and other places in the market.

- In 1968–1969, the "Hong Kong flu" pandemic killed approximately thirty-four thousand people in the United States.

- A rubella epidemic in 1964 infected 12.5 million people in the United States, killing infants by the thousands.

- In 1881 French chemist and microbiologist Louis Pasteur developed the first live-virus vaccine (against rabies).

Are Vaccines Safe?

In March 2011 in Japan, four children between the ages of three months and two years died shortly after receiving a vaccine called Prevnar, intended to protect against pneumococcal bacteria. Three of the children had also received a shot of the ActHIB vaccine against haemophilus influenza type b (Hib). Some of the children had also gotten other childhood vaccinations later that same day, but the only commonality among all four was Prevnar. As a result, the media began questioning the safety of the vaccine, and many parents wondered whether it was really necessary.

Both pneumococcal bacteria and Hib can cause serious infections, including pneumonia and meningitis. According to the CDC, in each year before the Hib vaccine was available, about twenty thousand US children under age five contracted a severe case of the infection, and nearly one thousand died from it. The CDC also reports that 5 percent of children under age five who contract meningitis die from it, and of those who survive, some are left deaf or blind.

Vaccinations have dramatically reduced the number of children contracting these diseases. Infants between the ages of two months and fifteen months typically receive four doses of Prevnar, and according to New York pediatrician Alanna Levine, "We've seen a vast decrease in pneumococcal infections once we started using Prevnar and avoided a lot of illness in children." She has seen no side effects from the vaccine except for a fever and/or rash and believes that the vaccine "has a good safety profile."[13]

Not Enough Tests

Despite these and other good reports about the vaccine, Japanese officials decided to suspend the use of Prevnar until a panel of experts at Japan's health ministry could investigate the situation. Just three weeks later they declared that there was no direct link between the deaths and either Prevnar or ActHIB. This kind of speed angers anti-vaccinationists, who believe that not enough resources are put into studying possible vaccine-related problems.

Anti-vaccinationists also believe that not enough testing is

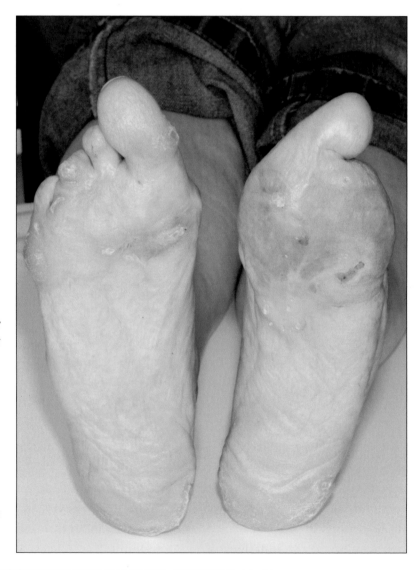

Impaired blood circulation caused by meningitis can require amputation of the toes (pictured). A vaccine for pneumococcal bacteria, an infection that can cause meningitis, was implicated in childhood deaths in Japan in 2011. An investigation found no direct link between the vaccine and the deaths.

done to determine the safety of new vaccines before they enter the marketplace. Prior to the FDA's approval of Prevnar for widespread use, for example, researchers tested the vaccine on only about eighteen thousand children. An additional sixty-five thousand nine hundred trials on children were done after approval, and another seventy-four hundred children were involved in trials in order to gain approval for a new version of the vaccine in 2010.

Federal officials are confident that these numbers are high enough to provide an accurate statistical picture of the vaccine's risk to the public, but anti-vaccinationists strongly disagree. For example, the Elizabeth Birt Center for Autism Law and Advocacy (EBCALA), which advocates for parents of children with autism, complains that the government has done little to investigate the connection between vaccinations and the onset of autism. The organization says,

> *"At this point, we largely know the benefits of vaccines, but the research on their potential risks is grossly inadequate."*[14]
>
> — The Elizabeth Birt Center for Autism Law and Advocacy.

> At this point, we largely know the benefits of vaccines, but the research on their potential risks is grossly inadequate. For years, advocates have asked that the government perform a large study of fully-vaccinated children compared to unvaccinated controls to assess their total health and to compare autism rates in the two populations. The standard response to our request has been silence.[14]

Indeed, the federal government has been unwilling to devote funds to studying a variety of possible connections between certain vaccines and certain health problems, and many people concerned about vaccine safety say that this is irresponsible. For example, microbiologist Howard Urnovitz, founder of the Chronic Illness Research Foundation in Berkeley, California, complains that federal officials cannot keep claiming there is no evidence that vaccines cause chronic illnesses when "they won't fund any research in that area. If you don't look for something, you won't find it."[15]

Others counter that the success of vaccines like Prevnar and ActHIB prove that the government's approach to testing is adequate. Over 360 million doses of Prevnar have been administered

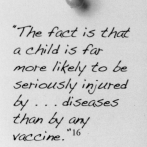
in more than 100 countries since its approval, and over 200 million doses of ActHIB have been administered in over 120 countries, and neither appears to have caused any serious problems. Other vaccines have been administered just as successfully, and many health experts argue that any problems caused by a vaccine must be considered with the risks of disease in mind. No vaccine is 100 percent safe, but as the CDC points out, "The fact is that a child is far more likely to be seriously injured by . . . diseases than by any vaccine. While any serious injury or death caused by vaccines is too many, it is also clear that the benefits of vaccination greatly outweigh the slight risk, and that many, many more injuries and deaths would occur without vaccinations."[16]

Few Side Effects

To monitor vaccine safety, the CDC and the FDA cosponsor a national vaccine safety surveillance program, the Vaccine Adverse Event Reporting System (VAERS). Under this system, these agencies collect information about possible side effects and other problems related to the administration of vaccines that have already been licensed for use in the United States. Because of the program's monitoring, the CDC says, "Vaccines are actually very safe, despite implications to the contrary in many anti-vaccine publications." The agency further reports,

> Most vaccine adverse events are minor and temporary, such as a sore arm or mild fever. . . . More serious adverse events occur rarely (on the order of one per thousands to one per millions of doses), and some are so rare that risk cannot be accurately assessed. As for vaccines causing death, again so few deaths can plausibly be attributed to vaccines that it is hard to assess the risk statistically.[17]

Causation Versus Coincidence

Health experts use the term "adverse event" to refer to a problem linked to the vaccine only by timing. That is, the event is something bad that happens shortly after the vaccination, and whether the event was caused by the vaccine or merely occurred at that time by coincidence is often unclear. As National Network for Immunization Information (NNII), an information clearinghouse, notes: "Because something happened at about the same time that a vaccine was given does not mean that the vaccine caused the problem."[18] Indeed, in compiling reports of adverse events, VAERS does not judge whether a particular vaccine is causing the problems being reported.

The job of attempting to rule out causation falls on government and pharmaceutical company researchers, who typically take a multipronged approach to studying an adverse event. Some of the researchers work to determine whether more cases of the adverse event have occurred than those already reported. Others conduct epidemiological studies to look at whether people who are unvaccinated are experiencing the same problem as those who have been vaccinated, which might suggest that something other than the vaccine is causing the problem. Still others study the vaccine itself, trying to determine whether some aspect of the vaccine might be causing adverse events.

Even after these exhaustive studies, researchers often are unable to prove that the vaccine could not possibly have caused the adverse event. More typically, their official conclusion is that the evidence does not support causation, which means that the vaccine is highly unlikely to have caused the event. In some countries, however, officials will declare a vaccine unsafe without such proof if the number of reported incidents is particularly high. For example, Finland and Sweden saw a dramatic rise in cases of narcolepsy—a disorder characterized by sudden attacks of deep sleep—among young people after mass vaccinations against the swine flu in 2009. Although studies on the connection between the vaccine and narcolepsy were typically inconclusive, both governments took responsibility for the narcolepsy cases and compensated the families of victims.

"Because something happened at about the same time that a vaccine was given does not mean that the vaccine caused the problem."[18]

— National Network for Immunization Information.

Childhood Problems

Narcolepsy can first present itself in childhood even when no flu shot has been given. In fact, many developmental problems are first diagnosed in childhood regardless of whether the victims have had vaccinations. For example, asthma affects as many as 10 to 12 percent of children in the United States, and most of these children show symptoms of this disorder by age five. Therefore, for asthma to coincidentally surface right after a childhood vaccination would not be a rare occurrence. Similarly, seizure disorders such as epilepsy are often diagnosed in childhood, so if a child had a seizure after a whooping cough shot, for example, this would not necessarily mean the shot was to blame. As Paul A. Offit, an expert on vaccination history, explains:

> Every year in the United States, in England, and throughout the world, children suffer epilepsy and mental retardation; this has been true for centuries, well before the pertussis vaccine was invented. Also, symptoms of epilepsy and retardation often occur in the first year of life, the same time that children are receiving three doses of the vaccine. Given the widespread use of pertussis vaccine, most children destined to develop seizures or mental retardation anyway would likely have received it, some within the previous twenty-four or forty-eight hours.[19]

Vaccine refusers have blamed the whooping cough vaccine for causing epilepsy. They have also blamed the hepatitis B vaccine for causing asthma because it includes an ingredient known to cause breathing problems independent of the vaccine. Specifically, the vaccine is made using baker's yeast, yeast proteins remain in the final product, and exposure to yeast is known to affect breathing in some people. In fact, some people are so allergic to yeast that the resulting breathing problems become life-threatening.

Vaccine Production

Some people have suggested that yeast be eliminated from the process of making hepatitis B vaccine. But the reason for the yeast's

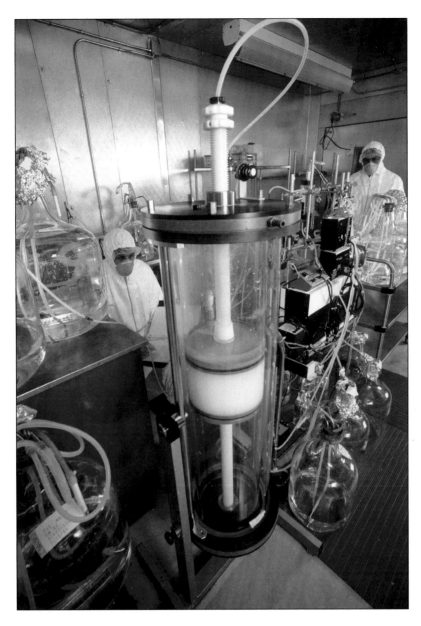

Hepatitis B vaccine production (pictured) involves genetic engineering and yeast cultures. Experts say the use of yeast in place of human blood plasma has improved the safety of this vaccine.

presence has to do with vaccine safety. Before yeast was employed, the vaccine was made using human plasma (the fluid portion of blood) infected with hepatitis B, and the antigens taken from the plasma had to be purified to make sure they were freed of live virus. Otherwise the vaccination could give recipients a contagious case of the disease. But in the 1980s scientists discovered they could create a recombinant version of the vaccine, which means the vaccine is produced through genetic engineering rather than the use of infected plasma. Vaccine manufacturers clone a portion of the hepatitis B virus gene into yeast, culture the yeast so that the material grows, and then use the yeast cultures to produce the vaccine.

Other vaccines are still produced using live viruses. They contain a small amount of the virus, weakened so that a recipient with a healthy immune system will not develop symptoms of the disease. (Therefore people with weakened immune systems cannot get such vaccinations.) The advantage to live-virus vaccines, which include those against measles, mumps, rubella, and chicken pox, is that they are so effective at triggering the body's immune response that far fewer doses are required in comparison with vaccines containing inactivated viruses. However, inactivated vaccines, such as those against pertussis, influenza, and polio (which comes in a live-virus version as well), are unable to cause the diseases they are intended to prevent because they use dead or killed viruses or bacteria to develop the body's immune response.

In addition to the agent of the disease, vaccine production also requires substances that help this agent grow and thrive during the development process. The polio virus, for example, is multiplied through the use of monkey kidney cells in a culture nourished by calf serum (a protein-rich liquid in blood). Measles and mumps viruses are nourished in cultures of chicken embryo cells, while rubella is nourished in human lung cells. As with yeast, residuals of these processes can be left behind in the final product. For example, vaccines made using chicken embryos will retain egg proteins, which means that someone who is allergic to eggs cannot be injected with those vaccines.

Additives and Preservatives

Vaccines also have additives such as formaldehyde, which is commonly used in embalming the dead. Formaldehyde eliminates the potentially harmful effects of bacterial toxins used in the production of vaccines. In vaccines produced using viruses, formaldehyde prevents those viruses from replicating, or multiplying. Human serum albumin (proteins filtered out of donated blood)

Doses

The number of shots required to immunize a person against a disease varies according to the disease and how the vaccine against that disease is made. Shots that employ live viruses to trigger an immune response, such as live-virus vaccines for chicken pox, mumps, measles, and rubella, typically require only one shot in childhood and then a booster shot a certain number of years later. Other vaccinations—the majority—require a series of shots, each of which provides a portion of the immune response necessary to fight the disease. According to Robert W. Sears in the 2011 edition of his book *The Vaccine Book*, when a vaccine is given in a series, the first shot provides 50 percent immunity, the second an additional 25 percent immunity, and by the third dose the recipient has approximately a 90 percent immunity to the disease being vaccinated against. Some of these vaccinations also require a fourth dose and/or a booster shot a year or more after the third dose in order to maintain this level of immunity.

is added to help stabilize live viruses in a vaccine. Aluminum salts are added to certain vaccines (but none of them live-virus) as a way to improve the body's immune response. Substances added to make vaccines work better are called adjuvants, and they typically lessen the number of doses of the vaccine required to achieve full immunization. Vaccines can also include preservatives, such as 2-phenoxyethanol, that prevent bacteria or fungi from contaminating the vaccine.

All of these additives and preservatives have come under fire from anti-vaccinationists, who believe such substances are toxic. But defenders of the practice say that these substances are not used in significant enough amounts to cause harm and that they already get into the human body in other ways. For example, aluminum occurs naturally in air, food, and water, and it is also added to certain foods like self-rising flour and infant formula. But except in people with kidney problems, it is flushed from the body relatively quickly, and no evidence of it harming anyone has surfaced during its decades of use. Formaldehyde also occurs naturally and does not seem to have caused problems. In fact, Paul Gallagher, an Australian skeptic who blogs about health-related issues, says, "Bemoaning formaldehyde exposure is as outrageous as it is ridiculous. A backyard BBQ burning old wood off-cuts or timber fixtures would produce many thousands of times that of a lifetime of vaccination. It's typical misrepresentation of how much dose makes a poison."[20]

Mercury

Many arguments related to vaccine safety revolve around what amount causes toxicity. People on both sides of vaccine issues agree that most medicines become poisons if administered in excessive doses. But what constitutes excessive?

One vaccine preservative involved in disputes over how much is too much is thimerosal, a powdered form of the metallic element mercury. When it was first added to vaccines in the 1930s, no one knew that in high amounts mercury can cause serious mental and developmental problems in children and mentally impair adults or increase their risk of heart attack. Even after evidence of this came to light, however, health experts continued to insist that the levels of mercury in vaccines were so low they would not cause any problems.

Over time, however, officials grew concerned that this was no longer the case, because as the number of recommended vaccinations grew, so too did the exposure to mercury-including shots. In fact, in one round of shots at a single check-up, a baby could get as much as eighty times more than the highest amount of mercury considered safe. Consequently, in 1999 the CDC, American Academy of Pediatrics, and FDA all called for the removal of thimerosal from all childhood vaccines, while insisting that this measure was purely precautionary.

By the end of 2002 at least one brand of every childhood vaccine was offered in a mercury-free version, and gradually many of the offerings containing mercury disappeared altogether. Some for-

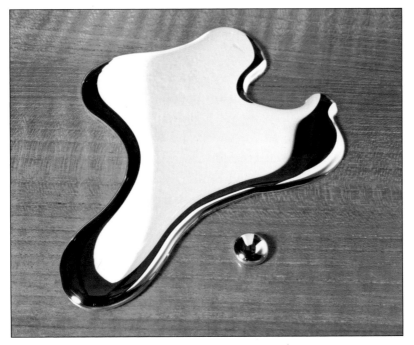

Until 1999 many vaccines contained a powdered form of mercury as a preservative. Contact with large amounts of mercury, shown here in liquid form, can result in mental and developmental problems in children.

mulations of the flu vaccine still contain thimerosal, though. Some experts say that these shots are safe because people do not get much mercury from just one shot. In fact, some experts have estimated that each dose of the vaccine contains no more than the amount of mercury in a six-ounce can of tuna fish. Nonetheless, pediatrician Robert W. Sears, an expert on immunization, recommends that skipping a flu shot is better than getting one with mercury in it.

Sears explains that he is basing this recommendation on a risk-benefit analysis. He reports that in the United States the number of deaths from the flu among children of all ages is usually less than one hundred per year, a very small number given the US population. Therefore, he says, "While flu fatalities may be preventable with the vaccine, you shouldn't live in fear that it's going to sweep through your community, killing children left and right." On the other hand, he reports, no one knows just how damaging mercury can be. He says: "We've known for decades that mercury is toxic to the brain and body tissues. But whether or not the amount in vaccines is enough to cause damage is still up in the air. Some research shows there is enough evidence of harm; other studies have found there is not enough proof that the mercury in vaccines is dangerous. However, no study has yet to prove for certain that this mercury is safe."[21]

Nonetheless, most experts do not recommend skipping a vaccination, even if the risk of contracting the disease targeted by the vaccine is small. As the CDC notes: "Remember, vaccines are continually monitored for safety, and like any medication, vaccines can cause side effects. However, a decision not to immunize a child also involves risk and could put the child and others who come into contact with him or her at risk of contracting a potentially deadly disease."[22]

Injecting Germs

Health officials also reject Sears's suggestion that childhood vaccinations be spaced out so that young people's immune systems are not exposed to too many vaccines in a short period. Sears believes that not enough research has been done to see whether the immune system can tolerate being stimulated to fight so many diseases at once. He contends that no studies have examined whether injecting foreign substances directly into the bloodstream is as safe as the natural way the body encounters such substances: through eating, drinking, and breathing. These processes allow the gastrointestinal and respiratory tracts to assault foreign substances before they reach the bloodstream. Consequently Sears suspects that injection carries more risk than natural exposure to germs because "our bodies were not designed to handle direct, internal germ exposure as easily. This is why we use sterile techniques during surgery and invasive medical procedures."[23] To him, this is another reason to avoid bombarding the body with many vaccinations within a short time period.

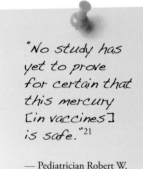

"No study has yet to prove for certain that this mercury [in vaccines] is safe."[21]

— Pediatrician Robert W. Sears.

But other experts argue that delaying vaccinations is even more dangerous to the immune system, because it increases the risk of disease. For example, the Vaccine Education Center at the Children's Hospital of Philadelphia says, "Delaying vaccines will only increase the time during which children are liable to catch

Vaccine Roulette

The 1982 national broadcast of an hour-long documentary entitled *DPT: Vaccine Roulette* did much to fuel anti-vaccination sentiments in the United States. Written and produced by NBC television correspondent Lea Thompson for WRC-TV in Washington, DC, this program suggested that the pertussis portion of the DPT (diphtheria, pertussis, tetanus) vaccination could cause brain damage, and it showed children who had become permanently disabled shortly after receiving a DPT shot. The scenes of these children were heart-wrenching, and in talking about the dangers of the whooping cough vaccine the documentary minimized the seriousness of whooping cough, leaving many viewers to question why the vaccine was necessary. Others who watched the program and had a child with brain injuries became convinced that these injuries had been caused by the vaccine. Among them was Barbara Loe Fisher, one of the leaders of the anti-vaccination movement in America, who cofounded the nonprofit charity National Vaccine Information Center (NVIC) for parents of such children in 1982 and wrote a book condemning the DPT vaccination, *DPT: A Shot in the Dark*, in 1985.

vaccine-preventable diseases. Certain diseases, such as whooping cough and pneumococcus, still occur commonly in the United States. . . . [Delaying vaccines] will only increase the child's chance of suffering a severe and potentially fatal infection."[24]

Not all infections are equally damaging, however. For this reason, some health professionals advise people concerned about vaccines to consider the risk-benefit ratios of each vaccine separately rather than judge the safety of vaccination as a whole. For example, the National Vaccine Information Center (NVIC) advises parents to evaluate a vaccination in the same way as any other medical procedure that "carries a risk of injury of death," saying, "It is your responsibility to become educated about the benefits and risks of vaccines in order to make the most informed, responsible vaccination decisions."[25] But as others note, a decision to reject a particular vaccination is difficult to implement wherever mandated vaccination programs do not allow people to pick and choose which ones of the mandated vaccines they want to have. Therefore anti-vaccinationists fight to eliminate any vaccine they deem too risky from such programs.

Facts

- In January 2000, US health experts stopped recommending the use of the oral polio vaccine because it was causing at least ten cases of polio a year.

- According to Paul A. Offit, an expert in vaccination issues, since 1999 the percentage of unvaccinated young people has more than doubled.

- Studies in Japan in the late 1970s and early 1980s showed that delaying DPT shots until children were the age of two resulted in an 85 to 90 percent reduction in cases of serious harm or death associated with the vaccine.

- Booster shots for measles were not added to immunization schedules in the United States until 1994; in Japan they were not added until 2006.

- Between 1992 and 2008 the state of Minnesota typically had no more than two cases of haemophilis influenza type B (Hib) a year, but in 2008 five children contracted the disease and one died because they had not been sufficiently immunized.

Should the HPV Vaccination Be Required?

I n 2007 Texas governor Rick Perry signed an executive order requiring that all girls entering the sixth grade in his state be inoculated against the human papillomavirus (HPV), a sexually transmitted virus that can cause cervical cancer. He was the first governor in the United States to mandate this vaccination, which requires three doses of vaccine to be effective. Perry justified this action by emphasizing the seriousness of HPV infections, but the order also included a provision allowing girls to be exempt from the vaccine if their parents filed a formal objection.

According to the CDC, there are roughly 6.2 million cases of HPV infection in the United States per year, and at least half of all Americans will contract the virus sometime in their lives. In fact, 80 percent of American women are infected by age fifty. There is no treatment that will eliminate the virus in an infected person. However, of the many strains of HPV in existence, more than half go away on their own without causing any health problems. In addition, only a few strains cause cervical cancer. Still, the disease is serious. In the United States nearly ten thousand women are diagnosed with cervical cancer each year, and thirty-seven hundred a year die of it.

Nonetheless, many Texans objected to Perry's vaccine mandate, and they had several reasons for their objections. The media initially focused on the fact that the vaccine's manufacturer,

Merck, had donated money to Perry's political campaign, and his friend, political supporter, and former chief of staff Mike Toomey was a lobbyist who worked for Merck. Perry's political opponents used these connections as a way to attack both him and the mandate, suggesting it was born out of money concerns rather than health concerns. These attacks and others led the Texas legislature to overrule Perry's order.

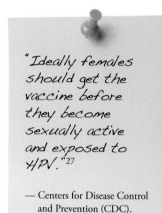

"Ideally females should get the vaccine before they become sexually active and exposed to HPV."[27]

— Centers for Disease Control and Prevention (CDC).

Immediately afterward, Perry defended his mandate by arguing that it had been necessary for the public good. "I challenge legislators to look these women in the eyes and tell them," he said, "'We could have prevented this disease for your daughters and granddaughters, but we just didn't have the gumption to address all the misguided and misleading political rhetoric.'" Later, however, Perry called the mandate "a mistake," and in August 2011 he said, "The fact of the matter is that I didn't do my research well enough to understand that we needed to have a substantial conversation with our citizenry"[26] before enacting the new mandate.

Too Young?

The conversation that many Texas parents wanted to have was about morals and choice rather than politics. When the idea of mandating the vaccine was introduced, these parents questioned why girls so young would have to be vaccinated for a sexually transmitted disease. They also argued that expressing approval of such a vaccine would be sending a message to girls that having sex at a young age is okay. Many parents wanted the choice to be able to say that it is not okay and therefore getting the vaccine is not okay.

The makers of the two HPV vaccines currently on the market—Gardasil, made by Merck, and Cervarix, made by GlaxoSmithKlein—have explained that the vaccine works best if it is given to girls before they become sexually active. (Gardasil is recommended for girls as young as ten, Cervarix for girls as young as eleven, and both are also recommend for males as young as nine to protect them against some types of genital warts.) The CDC elaborates, "Ideally females should get the vaccine before they be-

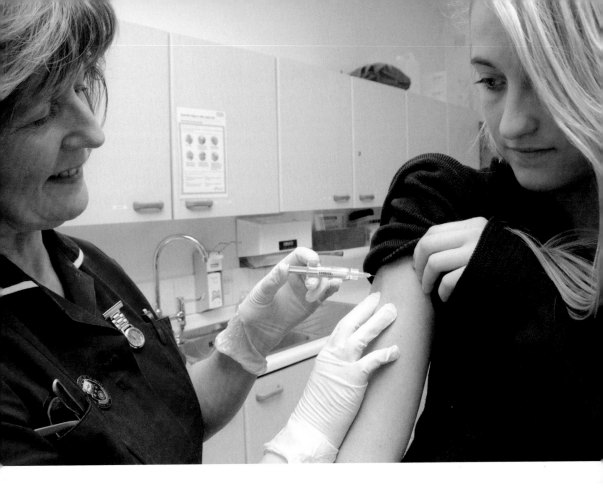

come sexually active and exposed to HPV. Females who are sexually active may also benefit from vaccination, but they may get less benefit. This is because they may have already been exposed to one or more of the HPV types targeted by the vaccines."[27]

Surveys indicate that less than 50 percent of parents are willing to vaccinate a 12-year-old girl against HPV, whereas roughly 70 to 90 percent cited an age within the years 15 to 18 as the point where they would find the vaccine appropriate. However, according to the Guttmacher Institute, an organization that conducts research and disseminates information regarding reproductive health worldwide, 13 percent of American teens have had sex by the age of 15, and 70 percent have had sex by the age of 19. Moreover, other researchers have found that among sexually active teens aged 13 to 21, 70 percent showed signs of an HPV infection occurring within months after starting to have sex.

A teenager is vaccinated against HPV, a sexually transmitted virus that can cause cervical cancer. To be effective, the vaccine must be given before a girl becomes sexually active. The vaccine has been characterized as prudent protection against a deadly disease but also as implied permission to become sexually active.

Encouraging Promiscuity?

Given these statistics, health experts say that it is safer, in terms of disease risk, to vaccinate girls as young as possible. But some people believe that giving young people access to anything that makes sex safer will encourage them to have sex. For example, shortly after the FDA approved Gardasil, Reginald Finger, a physician prominent among conservative Christian groups, commented that promoting the vaccine as making sex safer undermines abstinence-only teaching. He worries that once girls are vaccinated against HPV they will no longer consider sex off limits.

However, according to the National Survey of Family Growth (NSFG), an agency that researches teenage sexual behavior, the most common reasons for youth to engage in or not engage in sex have nothing to do with HPV. The main reasons that teens become sexually active are peer pressure and the use of alcohol or drugs. The main reasons that teens choose not to have sex are fear of pregnancy and of getting sexually transmitted diseases (STDs) such as herpes or gonorrhea. Author Meghan O'Rourke, in commenting on this issue for *Slate* magazine, says that many teens would be far more concerned with other STDs than with HPV. She explains, "HPV is hardly a major deterrent to kids who might be squeamish about STDs, since it has few short-term effects and cervical cancer usually takes years to develop. Adolescents have a hard enough time thinking about next week, let alone a decade from now. They're more likely to be worried about the immediate effect of herpes, gonorrhea, or syphilis, or even AIDS, which is still more prevalent than cervical cancer."[28]

Knowing Its Purpose

Most US children are already given a vaccine related to an STD: hepatitis B. This virus is transmitted via bodily fluids, including those associated with sexual contact, and it can cause a serious liver disease. Therefore nearly 90 percent of all children in the United States receive the mandated hepatitis vaccine by the time they are nineteen months old—and many experts have suggested that much of the controversy over the HPV vaccine would have been

Shots Without Permission

On January 30, 2012, a fourteen-year-old girl in Detroit, Michigan, was pulled out of class by the school nurse and sent to a clinic affiliated with her private school, the Marcus Garvey Academy. She then received vaccinations for hepatitis A, influenza, meningitis, and HPV (Gardasil) without the knowledge or permission of her mother. The mother, Sighle Kinney, was outraged when she learned about this violation of her wishes. A week later the girl developed a rash on her arms that soon spread to other parts of her body, and Kinney subsequently went to ABC News with her story. In the ABC report Kinney made it clear that she was opposed to the HPV vaccine and that in addition to not giving permission for the shot, she had previously signed a school document refusing all medical treatment for her daughter except in a life-or-death emergency. Kinney also questioned why the school would allow a school nurse to pull a student out of class and send her to a medical clinic without contacting a parent first, and many parents shared her anger that this had occurred. The school has declined to comment on the situation, citing its need to maintain student confidentiality. It encouraged the girl's mother to discuss her daughter's health needs with the clinic that gave the shots. This statement made some people wonder whether there might be more to the girl's story than what she told her mother.

avoided if it could be administered to children that young as part of regular mandated childhood vaccination.

In other words, some believe that resistance to HPV is based on the fact that recipients of the vaccine are aware of its purpose. However, surveys have shown that teens generally have such a low awareness of HPV that many do not even associate it with sex.

And as Nancy Gibbs, who has reported on the issue for *Time* magazine, notes, adults need not point out this connection. She says:

> There may well be parents who are reluctant to give their nine-year-old in pigtails a vaccine against a sexually transmitted disease, that the very idea makes them uncomfortable. But . . . most doctors won't declare, as they administer the vaccine, "There! Now when you go out and have promiscuous, unprotected intercourse with strangers, at least there is one less sexually transmitted disease to worry about." I think they're much more likely to say, "This will only hurt for a second."[29]

In the case of older teens, Gibbs adds, "Even if, as they got older, girls did understand somehow what the vaccine was protecting them against, surely the messages parents send to them every day and over the years—about respect, responsibility, judgment and the boundaries of appropriate sexual behavior—count for more than the implicit suggestion of a single vaccine."[30]

Physician Shobha S. Krishnan shares this view. Moreover, she suggests that parents who allow their daughters to receive the vaccination can use it as an opportunity to discuss not only sex but health. She says, "There is no reason why parents cannot, without any hypocrisy, inform their daughters that the vaccine is not a green light for them to immediately have sex. Rather, it is a strong message that . . . their parents care about their health, and that it's important to take proactive steps to become a healthy adult."[31]

In fact, the vaccine does not appear to make sexually active girls more promiscuous. That is, after receiving the vaccine, a girl who has already had sex does not typically increase her sexual activity. This was the conclusion of an NSFG study released in December 2011 involving girls aged fifteen to twenty-four who had been vaccinated against HPV and understood the vaccine's connection to the sexually transmitted disease. The study also found that girls continued to

"There is no reason why parents cannot, without any hypocrisy, inform their daughters that the vaccine is not a green light for them to immediately have sex."[31]

— Physician and parent Shobha S. Krishnan.

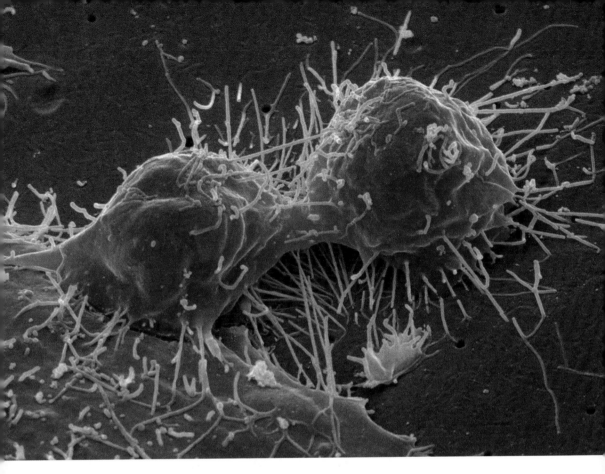

use condoms at the same rate, thereby remaining careful to protect themselves from unwanted pregnancies and from other sexually transmitted diseases.

Nonetheless, some of those opposed to vaccinating teens against HPV have suggested that only girls who are already sexually active need the shot. For example, George Warren, the father of a nine-year-old girl in California, says of his daughter, "She's not gonna need it [the shot]. I'm a good parent. I tell her what's right and wrong."[32] And in 2007, as a Republican state senator of California, George Runner questioned the need to mandate a vaccine that was tied to "personal choices,"[33] implying that only the promiscuous would need protection against cervical cancer.

Personal Choice

Other opponents to HPV mandates emphasize a different type of choice: that of parents to decide whether they want their children

Cervical cancer, which can be caused by HPV, is one of the most common cancers affecting women. A cervical cancer cell is shown in a colored scanning electron micrograph.

to have the vaccination. In fact, some opponents make a clear distinction between the issue of whether the vaccine is a good thing and the issue of whether it should be mandated. Linda Klepacki works on issues related to sexual health for Focus on the Family—a conservative Christian group often criticized for its opposition to the HPV vaccine. Klepacki says her organization does not actually oppose the vaccine. "This is an awesome vaccine. It could prevent millions of deaths around the world. We support this vaccine. We see it as an extremely important medical breakthrough. To read those headlines saying we're against this is really disconcerting."[34]

What Focus on the Family opposes, says Klepacki, is making the vaccine mandatory. Her organization believes that parents should decide whether to vaccinate their daughters—and when. "This is a disease you don't catch by sneezing or coughing. It's linked to a behavior. You don't contract HPV by sitting in a classroom. So this is a different issue [than already mandated childhood vaccinations]. . . . We want it to be out of the government's hands and in the parents' hands, because this is a sexually transmitted infection."[35]

Others, however, note that without mandates, far fewer people get a vaccine, and HPV is so widespread in the population that millions of doses are necessary to combat its spread. O'Rourke, for example, complains that while people opposed to the vaccine are fighting mandates, they are missing "the chance to eradicate the HPV virus and its associated cancers from the lives of young Americans."[36] Similarly, Krishnan says, "As a mother, I can understand why many parents are concerned about this issue and put off vaccinating their daughters. However, in addition to being a mother, I am a physician, and I therefore believe that by putting off vaccination, we effectively strip our daughters from their chances of protecting themselves from two major cancer-causing HPV types."[37]

Pap Smears

But is the vaccine really necessary to fight cervical cancer? Some people say it is not, as indicated by death statistics. According to the National Institutes of Health, as of January 2012 only three per one hundred thousand people in the United States die of cervical cancer. Many experts believe the low rate can be attributed to early detection and treatment made possible by routine Pap tests. A Pap (Papanicolaou) test is a cervical cancer screening whereby cells collected from the cervix are examined to see whether they are noncancerous, premalignant (about to become cancerous), or malignant (cancerous). Introduced in the 1940s and promoted by the American Cancer Society in 1945, the Pap test did not become a routine part of women's health exams in the United States until the 1960s. Since that time cervical cancer rates among US women have dropped by 70 percent. At the same time, when women neglect to get their routine Pap tests or do not have the money for them, their risk of contracting cervical cancer rises. In fact, the CDC has found that most women diagnosed with cervical cancer in the United States have never had a Pap test or have not had one in over five years.

Health experts point to these statistics as proof that Pap screenings alone are enough to prevent cervical cancer. Consequently the CDC recommends that even women who have had the HPV vaccination should get Pap tests, since the HPV vaccine does not combat all forms of the HPV virus. Gardasil protects against only four of the more than one hundred types of HPV, while Cervarix protects against only two. However, proponents of the vaccine point out that if women fail to get their Pap tests, they become vulnerable to all HPVs, whereas those who had earlier received the vaccine would at least be protected against some HPVs.

Still, the National Cancer Institute has found that most high-risk HPV infections—that is, infections capable of causing cervical cancer—go away on their own without ever causing cancer. Studies have also shown that 90 percent of women clear HPVs from their bodies within two years of contracting them, whereupon the cervix gradually returns to normal. Anti-vaccine groups cite these facts to support their view that the HPV vaccine is unnecessary. One of the vaccine's most outspoken critics, Barbara Loe Fisher,

"This is an awesome vaccine. It could prevent millions of deaths around the world. We support this vaccine."[34]

— Linda Klepacki of the conservative Christian group Focus on the Family.

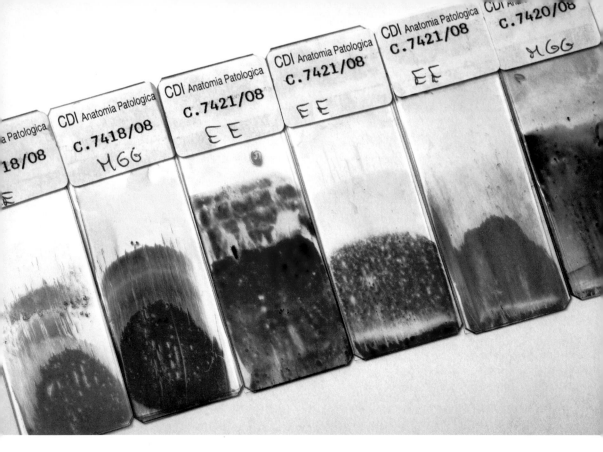

Cervical smear slides, obtained through routine Pap tests, are used to look for abnormalities that might indicate cancer. Pap screenings, done routinely, are an effective tool for preventing cervical cancer.

says that money is the primary motivator behind the campaign for the HPV vaccine. She contends that millions of young women are getting a vaccine they do not need because of heavy promotion by the manufacturer.

Dangerous?

Anti-vaccinationists also argue that the vaccine is too untried to be trusted. Approved for use in the United States in 2006–2007, the two versions of the vaccine were tested on about twenty thousand test subjects worldwide prior to reaching the marketplace, a number that experts believe is adequate but anti-vaccinationists do not. In either case, as of June 2012 more than 46 million doses of HPV vaccine had been distributed in the United States, and according to the CDC no serious health issues were associated with these doses or with those administered during testing. The CDC also says that the side effects reported so far have been mild—primarily fever, dizziness, nausea, and fainting right after vaccination.

However, Robert W. Sears reports that during initial testing of the vaccine, some worrisome problems did arise. In a study comparing a group vaccinated with HPV with a control group that did not receive the vaccine, females in the study group were significantly more likely to experience certain eye problems, thyroid problems, inflammatory bowel disease, multiple sclerosis, and arthritis. Males were more likely to experience arthritis and thyroid problems as well.

Adverse events also have been associated with the vaccine since it went on the market. For example, the CDC confirms that some young women have experienced blood clots in the heart, lungs, or legs after getting Gardasil. However, it adds that over 90 percent of these women had engaged in behavior that put them at greater risk of developing blood clots. (They smoked, for example, or took oral contraceptives.) Therefore the CDC has concluded that the blood clots were not caused by the Gardasil.

A Serious Disease

In arguments concerning the HPV vaccine, people often forget just how serious a disease cervical cancer can be. As an example of what sufferers often experience, the website of the Seattle Cancer Care Alliance provides the story of Elizabeth Records of Mercer Island, Washington, whose heavy menstrual periods in 2002 caused her to be concerned about her health. Finally she went to an emergency room, where doctors found a large tumor on her cervix that could not be removed surgically. After a diagnosis confirmed that the tumor was advanced cervical cancer, Records had radiation therapy to stop the bleeding. She then endured chemotherapy, external radiation, and internal radiation to destroy the cancer cells in her cervix during a year of aggressive treatments, but the cancer spread to her lungs. Surgeons were able to remove the tumor; Records's cancer has been in remission since that time.

The CDC has similarly dismissed claims that the HPV vaccine can increase the risk of developing GBS. From 2006 to 2008, thirty-six cases of GBS were reported after an HPV vaccination. Of these, 75 percent developed the disorder within six weeks, and 60 percent had received no other vaccine during that time or at the same time as their HPV vaccination. However, a study of these cases showed that the HPV vaccine was not necessarily to blame.

Says lead researcher Nizar Souayah, a neurologist with the University of Medicine and Dentistry of New Jersey, "Our results show that Guillain-Barré is not occurring more often after HPV vaccination than it does in the general population. However, the fact that most of these cases occurred within six weeks of vaccination does warrant careful monitoring for any additional cases and continued analysis."[38]

Nonetheless, in January 2012 a class-action lawsuit was filed in Australia against Merck by a young woman who began suffering from neurological problems after being injected with Gardasil. Specifically, after her first injection she suffered convulsions, experienced severe back and neck pain, and soon lost the ability to walk. Other women who have considered joining the lawsuit suffered strokes, paralysis, muscle pain, chronic fatigue, seizures, miscarriages, and other serious problems after getting a Gardasil injection. In addition, between May 2009 and September 2010 forty-two seemingly healthy young women died following Gardasil vaccinations. Anti-vaccine groups insist that this number proves causality, but others say the deaths merely happened to coincide with the vaccination, and close examination of these cases revealed other possible reasons for the deaths.

Another Way to Prevent HPV

Sears understands these concerns, but while he is a critic of some other vaccines, he says that HPV vaccine seems "a fairly good idea," adding, "It has the potential to decrease cervical cancer dramatically in our population if it works as well as it is hoped. If all preteens are vaccinated, eventually these common strains of HPV will stop circulating in our population and the rates of genital warts

"Teens and young adults who choose to delay sexual activity can safely defer the [HPV] vaccine."[40]

— Physician Robert W. Sears.

and cervical cancer should decrease for a while."[39] But Sears also notes that vaccination can only prevent four of the many strains of HPV, which means that vaccination cannot eliminate all HPVs, at least for the foreseeable future.

Moreover, Sears points out that "HPV disease (like hepatitis B disease) is virtually 100 percent preventable by our choices," explaining, "Public health officials would argue that every teen will choose to have sex with multiple people without considering the consequences, so there is risk for everyone and the vaccine should be given to every preteen. But teens do have other choices. Those who choose to have sex should be vaccinated. . . . Teens and young adults who choose to delay sexual activity can safely defer the vaccine."[40] This way, he suggests, young people can avoid the risks of the disease unless and until they face an actual risk of contracting HPV—and by that time, they might be old enough to make the decision about vaccination themselves, without having to rely on a parent's judgment. But experts counter that this ignores the fact that a teen's first sexual experience might not be planned, and that after that first sexual encounter it might already be too late to prevent HPV.

Facts

- As of July 2012 each dose of the HPV vaccine costs $130, which means the full series of shots costs $390, and not all insurance plans cover this cost.

- As of 2012 only Virginia and the District of Columbia had mandated an HPV vaccination, but eight states were considering similar legislation.

- Only 32 percent of teenage girls have received the complete three-dose series of the HPV.

- Most states require proof of all three doses of the hepatitis B vaccination for anyone entering day care, kindergarten, sixth grade, high school, or college.

CHAPTER FOUR

What Are the Consequences of Refusing Vaccinations?

In early 2012 health experts tracking the source of a measles outbreak in the United States discovered that it originated with two people traveling together to the Super Bowl game in Indianapolis, Indiana. On February 3, 2012, two days before the game, these individuals visited the Super Bowl Village, then a coffee shop, a restaurant, and a souvenir shop. Everywhere they went, according to officials, they exposed others to the risk of contracting measles, a highly contagious viral infection of the respiratory system that can cause encephalitis (an inflammation of the brain), pneumonia, and/or death.

However, the experts investigating the outbreak doubt the two travelers knew they were infected with anything more serious than a cold or flu. Measles begins with the same symptoms as these illnesses, and the telltale sign that the sufferer has measles instead—an angry red rash—does not appear for up to eight days after the coldlike symptoms have begun. Moreover, a person with the measles is the most contagious four days before the rash appears.

Only fourteen people are known to have contracted measles as a result of the Super Bowl event. All of them were from an area in Indiana where parents had been refusing to vaccinate their children against measles, and thirteen of the cases were within anti-vaccination families whose members socialized with each other. Health officials subsequently confirmed that thirteen of the victims had not received the MMR vaccination by choice.

Indiana's health commissioner, Gregory Larkin, therefore calls these cases "so significantly preventable."[41] Indeed, according to various studies, the measles vaccine is 95 percent effective in preventing the disease, and vaccination efforts have been so successful in the past that in 2000 measles was considered eradicated in the United States. This success is due largely to the fact that 90 percent

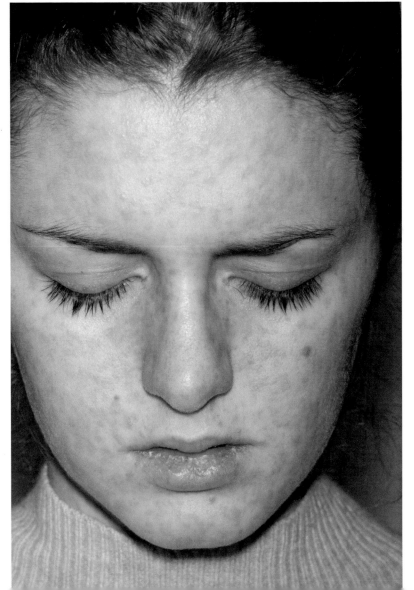

Initial symptoms of measles, a highly contagious disease, are similar to symptoms of a cold or flu. Eventually a red rash develops as can be seen on the face of a nineteen-year-old woman infected with measles.

of parents get their children immunized against childhood diseases, including measles—the likely reason that more people were not affected by the Super Bowl contagion.

Herd Immunity

Percentages are important when it comes to disease spread. This is because of the concept of herd immunity, which arose in the 1930s as a result of studies in how measles spread through communities. This idea suggests that individuals in a community who are not immune to a disease can be protected from contracting that disease by the immunity of those around them—their so-called herd. As a contagious disease is passed from person to person, the chain of transmission is broken if the next person the disease encounters is immune to it. The higher the number of immune people, the more chains are broken, and the less likely someone susceptible to the disease will be exposed to it.

Herd immunity is the justification behind allowing a certain number of vaccination exemptions. If the number of exempted people is sufficiently small in comparison to the size of the herd, disease spread is minimal. But as the number of unvaccinated people rises, herd immunity weakens, and the risk to the community rises accordingly. Family physician Stephanie Cave explains, "To achieve a high level of herd immunity, advocates of mass immunization strive for the highest vaccination rates possible with the hope that virtually everyone in the selected group will be protected from disease."[42]

Health experts are able to calculate the vaccination rate necessary to keep a disease from spreading within a population. The necessary percentage varies because diseases have different levels of contagion, but the number usually falls within 70 to 100 percent of the population. Based on this percentage, countries can set vaccination goals in an attempt to eradicate certain diseases within a group. For example, Brazil set a goal of vaccinating 70 million people from infancy to age thirty-nine against measles and as a result, in 2010 the World Health Organization declared that measles had been eradicated from the country.

"To achieve a high level of herd immunity, advocates of mass immunization strive for the highest vaccination rates possible with the hope that virtually everyone in the selected group will be protected from disease."[42]

— Family physician Stephanie Cave.

Natural Immunity

Vaccine proponents say that such successes depend on people who consider the good of others and society before they reject a vaccine, because maximum compliance to a vaccination program is vital to maintaining the overall health of the herd. As the World Health Assembly, a forum of the World Health Organization, has stated: "Vaccination is not simply a personal affair. Indeed, it is essentially a community matter, since the objective of most vaccination programmes is to produce a herd immunity."[43]

However, vaccine refusers believe that the only true immunity is natural immunity—immunity that develops naturally in the body after a person has contracted a disease and successfully fought it off. This belief is based on differences between the way the immune system responds to a disease as opposed to a vaccine. When someone develops an immunity to a disease by having had that disease, the immunity usually lasts a lifetime. This is not only because the immune system responds more dramatically while fighting off a disease, but because immunity is reinforced with each exposure to someone fighting off the disease. In other words, the immune are getting a natural "booster shot" from each new disease case in the community.

Also, a woman who is naturally immune to a disease passes antibodies against that disease to the fetus via the placenta. This does not occur when a mother has immunity to a disease only through vaccination. Therefore, according to the Vaccination Risk Awareness Network (VRAN), "most of today's babies are more vulnerable than babies of the pre-vaccine era."[44]

> "Most of today's babies are more vulnerable than babies of the pre-vaccine era."[44]
>
> — Vaccination Risk Awareness Network (VRAN).

A Healthier Herd

Vaccine refusers argue that this vulnerability is a reason to stop vaccinating. They do not think abandoning vaccination programs will weaken herd immunity because they do not think vaccine-provided herd immunity truly exists, especially since vaccines typically do not provide lifelong protection. For example, neurosurgeon Russell Blaylock, an expert on vaccines, says, "One of the grand lies of the vaccine program is the concept of 'herd immunity.' In fact, vaccines for most Americans decline to non-protective levels within 5 to 10 years of the vaccines. This means that for the vast majority of Americans, as well as others in the developed world, herd immunity doesn't exist and hasn't for over 60 years."[45]

Blaylock therefore argues that people should be allowed to contract and fight off diseases, although he adds that if vaccination programs are eliminated then people will have to take better care of their health so they can fight off infections effectively. Many anti-vaccinationists share this view, insisting that a healthier lifestyle will make vaccines unnecessary. For example, Jini Patel Thompson, a proponent of natural healing, argues that vaccines are unhealthy, that diseases can be eliminated without vaccines, and that the key to combating disease in the pre-vaccination era was "improved hygiene, better nutrition, clean drinking water, and improved sanitation." She adds: "Basically, as people's overall health and immune systems improved, they didn't get sick."[46]

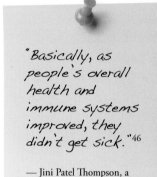

"Basically, as people's overall health and immune systems improved, they didn't get sick."[46]

— Jini Patel Thompson, a proponent of natural healing.

Serious Consequences

Unfortunately, Thompson is incorrect. People did get sick. In fact, many of them died from their diseases, and those who managed to survive were often left with permanent scars or disabilities that made their lives torturous. According to the Vaccine Education Center, "The price paid for immunity after natural infection might be pneumonia from chicken pox, mental retardation from *Haemophilus influenzae* type b (Hib), pneumonia from pneumococcus, birth defects from rubella, liver cancer from hepatitis B virus, or death from measles. Immunization with vaccines . . . does not extract such a high price for immunity."[47]

Vaccine proponents cannot understand why anyone would want to return to the days when diseases were allowed to run rampant. They also note that people like Thompson, who say that improving health keeps people from getting sick, are ignoring the fact that some people are unable to improve their health enough to fight off such serious diseases. Vaccine proponents also insist that immunity is immunity, whether it comes naturally or through a vaccine, and booster shots take care of the problem of immunity wearing off—as long as people get their booster shots. Otherwise they are putting at risk the most vulnerable members of society: infants and people with compromised immune systems.

In fact, because vaccine refusers put others in the community at risk, some pediatricians are refusing to accept unvaccinated children as patients. Surveys released in 2011 indicate that 20 to 30 percent of pediatricians have dismissed patients from their practice for refusing vaccines, usually after trying to change their minds about vaccinations. One such pediatrician, David Fenner, says vaccine refusers cannot be his patients because they cling to misinformation, which means "there are so many things we're not going to see eye-to-eye on."[48]

Foreign Influences

A common misconception is that because the United States has such a widespread vaccination program the chance of encountering someone with a contagious disease is almost zero. This might have been the case before international air travel was popularized in the mid-twentieth century, but the American "herd" now includes people from other countries. As *Slate* magazine columnist Amanda Marcotte notes, "In our modern era of plane travel, dense cities, and events like the Super Bowl, the average person has plenty of opportunities to inhale the germs of a large and diverse group of people—and take those germs further faster than ever before."[49]

Several recent outbreaks were caused by international travel. For example, in 2009–2010, over fifteen hundred people in New York and New Jersey were infected with mumps by an eleven-year-old boy who had traveled from the United States to the UK and back again. The main symptoms of mumps are fever and swelling of the salivary glands, but it can lead to inflammation of the brain, testicles, or ovaries. Ten to 20 percent of

"In our modern era of plane travel, dense cities, and events like the Super Bowl, the average person has plenty of opportunities to inhale the germs of a large and diverse group of people—and take those germs further faster than ever before."[49]

— Amanda Marcotte of *Slate* magazine.

people who have a contagious case of the mumps either never experience symptoms or do not develop symptoms for two to four months after becoming contagious. This was the case with the eleven-year-old boy, who had no idea (nor did his parents) that he was infecting others. However, his travels took place while the UK was in the midst of a mumps epidemic that ultimately infected over four thousand people. Similarly, in 2011 there were two hundred documented cases of measles in the United States—the most since 1996—and over 90 percent were triggered by infected visitors from abroad at a time when measles cases in Europe numbered thirty thousand.

International Events

Health experts report that such outbreaks have increased their worry over the possibility that the United States will be caught up in a pandemic of preventable diseases that, if the numbers of unvaccinated people continue to rise, could affect millions. One of the most worrisome outbreaks in terms of global implications involved measles cases traced to the 2010 Winter Olympics in Vancouver, Canada. People in British Columbia (BC), the province where Vancouver is located, began coming down with measles just nine days after the closing ceremonies. Eventually BC health officials saw eighty-five cases. Prior to the games, since 2002, measles in BC had amounted to only four cases a year.

Experts evaluating the situation discovered that most of the victims were young people who had partied at outdoor celebrations in downtown Vancouver. In addition, most of those who contracted the disease had either never been vaccinated as children or had not had a recommended booster shot as teenagers. A few babies who had not yet had their initial shots were also infected. About 20 percent of the victims were hospitalized because of their illness, and one had to be in the intensive care unit of the hospital.

Preventing outbreaks at such events is typically beyond the scope of health officials. "It's very difficult, if not impossible for public health officials to regulate that type of thing," reports William Moss of the Johns Hopkins Bloomberg School of Public Health.[50] Therefore, he says, attendees need to protect themselves

Spreading Disease

It takes only one unvaccinated person to introduce a disease into a community. For example, on January 13, 2008, an unvaccinated seven-year-old boy carried the measles virus from a vacation in Switzerland to his home in San Diego, California. The boy did not seem sick at the time, but nine days after arriving in California he developed what his parents thought was an ordinary cold. They sent him to school anyway, but when he seemed worse the next day, they took him to his doctor, whose waiting room was filled with other patients. The doctor then sent the boy to the hospital to have some tests, and while waiting for the results his parents took him home. Hours later, the boy's symptoms worsened and his parents took him to the hospital's emergency room, where he was finally diagnosed as being contagious with measles. Beginning on January 31, unvaccinated children, some of them infants, who had been near the boy began getting sick. One of these children carried the disease to Hawaii before coming down with symptoms, just as the boy who started the outbreak had carried it to California.

by getting vaccinated. In some cases, these vaccinations are mandated by the host country; Saudi Arabia, for example, has required polio vaccinations for attendees of certain gatherings in order to keep the country free of polio. But officials in Brazil have taken a different approach in preparation for hosting the 2014 World Cup. Brazil has mandated measles and rubella vaccinations for all workers who would come into contact with tourists at places like airports, hotels, and restaurants. These two diseases are being targeted because, thanks to an aggressive vaccination program, the only reported cases of measles (since 2002) and rubella (since 2008) have been among tourists who brought the diseases into the country.

Polio Spreads in Nigeria

Health experts say that Brazil is an example of how mandatory vaccinations can improve the health of a country. Conversely, they point to Nigeria as a cautionary tale of what can happen if too many people reject vaccination. Between 1996 and 2001, Nigeria was working with the World Health Organization (WHO) to eradicate polio, but today Nigeria is one of only three countries—along with Afghanistan and Pakistan—where polio is endemic. (An endemic disease is one that occurs regularly in a particular area.) Moreover, the spread of polio in Nigeria has affected other African countries. The disease has been reestablished in three countries that were previously polio-free, Angola, Chad, and Democratic Republic of the Congo, and in 2011 several more countries had outbreaks of the disease.

The WHO's goal since 1988 has been to rid the world of polio because, while other more deadly diseases exist, polio can cause lifelong suffering. In its most severe form it attacks the nervous system, which causes physical deformities, muscle damage, and paralysis. The disease can be spread by direct contact with throat secretions or infected stool, but in developing countries like Nigeria it is typically spread by the ingestion of food or drinking water that has been contaminated by the poor sanitary habits of people carrying the virus. (The virus occurs naturally only in humans.)

Given Nigeria's size and its many political conflicts and complexities, health experts have found it difficult to improve the country's sanitary conditions quickly enough to prevent the continuing spread of polio. A series of vaccination programs, however, has been so successful that in 2001 health experts said that they expected Nigeria to be polio-free by 2005. At this point they stepped up their vaccination efforts, which from the outset employed the live-virus form of the polio vaccine as a way to use the unsanitary conditions to their benefit. (When the live-virus vaccine is excreted it retains some potency, and if it ends up in drinking water due to poor hygiene, other people can be passively vaccinated.)

Unfortunately, a stronger push for vaccination resulted in stronger opposition from Nigerians suspicious of Western medi-

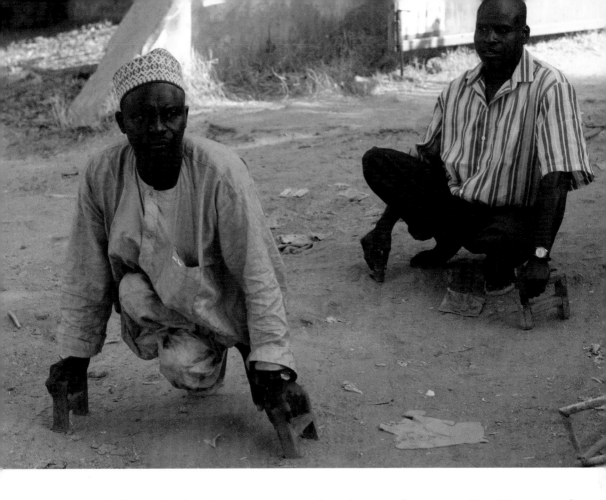

cine, and religious leaders began urging people to boycott the vaccine. Eventually the religious leaders' position was supported by political leaders in northern Nigeria, who then halted immunization efforts there. Jennifer G. Cooke and Farhar Tahir of the CSIS (Center for Strategic & International Studies) Global Health Policy Center, explain the thinking behind this decision:

> The north's relative isolation has to some extent fostered distrust and suspicion of external—particularly Western—interventions. As the polio campaign intensified, a host of rumors sprang up, some fueled by local imams [religious leaders] that the immunization effort was a Western plot to control or eliminate Muslim populations in the north by causing sterility or spreading the HIV virus. The fact that the vaccine was provided free of charge and distributed by

Two Nigerians who contracted polio and lost the use of their legs to the disease propel themselves through dusty streets. Nigeria experienced a huge resurgence of polio after that country's leaders halted a World Health Organization vaccination campaign there.

government health workers to even the most remote communities heightened suspicions, as parents wondered why medicine and medical services for far more common and deadly illnesses like malaria, cholera, and diarrheal disease were neither free nor readily accessible.[51]

The boycott dramatically reduced vaccinations, which in turn caused cases of polio to rise just as dramatically. (Measles and diphtheria cases increased as well, as anti-vaccination fervor spread.) Soon the situation in Nigeria spread beyond its borders. Roughly twenty countries were reinfected with polio ultimately traced to Nigeria, and by 2006 Nigeria was accounting for more than half of all polio cases worldwide. Consequently, Walter Orenstein, deputy director for the Gates Foundation's Global Health Program, says, "Polio is only a plane ride away from the United States. If we let our guard down, if our immunization coverage drops, there is certainly the possibility of a polio outbreak. Diphtheria could also come back. Any of them can."[52]

More Ages at Risk

The growing problem led Islamic leaders in other countries to convince Nigerian leaders to return to vaccination. As part of their effort to address suspicions about the vaccine, any polio vaccine used in Nigeria is now produced in Indonesia, where Muslims are in the majority, and vaccinations are again ongoing in Nigeria.

However, the gap in vaccination created by the boycott has been making it difficult for Nigeria and other parts of Africa to regain their footing in the fight against polio. Outbreaks continue to occur, such as one in the Congo in 2010–2011 that infected over ninety people. The Congo outbreaks and outbreaks during that same period in the central Asian country of Tajikistan—where religious leaders have also prevented vaccination—caused paralysis in hundreds of children and killed many adults.

Bruce Aylward, the head of WHO's Global Polio Eradication Initiative, reports that the death of so many adults from what has always been considered a childhood illness has affected the way health experts think about polio.

Many people had, for a long time, almost lied to themselves, saying that if eradication [of polio] failed it wouldn't really matter, that we could just continue with cases at a very low level. People are starting to understand that over time we are again going to have over a quarter of a million children paralysed every single year if [WHO's program to eradicate polio] fails. And it's not going to be a gradual creep back up that nobody notices, we could have serious backlashes in places that have long been polio-free, with tremendous mortality rates in adults.[53]

A College Requirement

College students are up to six times more likely to contract bacterial meningitis, a contagious infection spread like the common cold, and their risk of dying from the disease is five times higher than other age groups. Consequently many colleges now require students to be vaccinated against bacterial meningitis or to receive a booster shot if they were vaccinated more than five years before starting college. The state of Texas, for example, requires all college students under the age of thirty, even those living off campus, to get an initial vaccination or a booster shot unless they can provide a valid reason for exemption. The driving force behind this 2012 legislation was Patsy Schanbaum, whose daughter Jamie contracted meningitis while a student at the University of Texas at Austin in 2008. Jamie spent months in the hospital and lost most of her fingers and both legs to the disease, which can turn limbs gangrenous. Another young person from Austin, Alexander Reinis, died of bacterial meningitis in his dorm room in November 2011 while studying abroad in London. Reinis had initially been vaccinated six years earlier and had not received a booster shot.

Nonetheless, anti-vaccinationists maintain that instead of putting so much time, effort, and money into vaccination programs in developing countries, the same resources should be put into improving sanitary conditions in these countries, which they believe will eradicate diseases such as polio in a better, safer way.

Facts

- According to the US Centers for Disease Control and Prevention, only about half of all teenagers have received the meningococcal vaccine, which protects against bacterial infections that may lead to amputation of infected limbs and death.

- About 49 percent of all US adolescents received the recommended influenza vaccine during the 2010–2011 influenza season.

- Experts have determined that to prevent the spread of polio, 70 percent of the population needs to be immunized, whereas 90 percent of the population needs to be immunized against measles, because measles is more contagious than polio.

- Before the chicken pox vaccine was available, about ten thousand children a year were hospitalized and seventy died because of the disease.

Does Mandating Vaccines Violate People's Rights?

I n 2012 the Vermont Senate voted to eliminate the philosophical exemption from their state's mandatory vaccination law so that people could no longer cite personal beliefs as a reason for avoiding vaccination. However, the state House of Representatives voted against this change, arguing that a person should have the freedom to reject or delay a vaccine based on any kind of belief, not just a religious one. (The state was leaving its religious exemption in place.) As the two sides debated the issue, people began staging public protests for and against the law.

Among the law's opponents were the parents of seven-year-old Kaylynne Matten, who died in Vermont just four days after a routine flu shot in December 2011. Kaylynne seemed healthy when she was given the vaccination, and although a coroner later determined that her heart was inflamed—a condition called myocarditis that is usually caused by a virus—the influenza vaccine was not found in Kaylynne's heart. Therefore the coroner could not determine a cause of death. Still, her parents believe the flu shot killed her, and they did not want to be required to vaccinate their other children or leave them out of school.

At a rally against the Vermont law change, Kaylynne's mother, Nicole Matten, said, "Now, while we're grieving for our beautiful 7-year-old Kaylynne, we have to worry about our philosophical exemption being taken away from our other kids. It should be a parent's choice, this should be a free country."[54]

Another opponent of the law, the Vermont Coalition for Vaccine Choice, stated, "There is no need to allow the state to strip parents of their rights to make medical decisions for their own kids. Given that vaccines have known risks associated with them, it seems only prudent to continue the philosophical exemption."[55] In the end, to the dismay of many health experts, state lawmakers sided with this position and kept the philosophical exemption.

Freedom of Opinion

Such experts say that providing a philosophical rejection increases the unvaccinated percentage of the population to a dangerous level. In Vermont, for example, children are vaccinated at a rate 73 percent lower than the national average, and parents' use of the philosophical exemption is among the highest in the nation. Currently, twenty states offer this exemption, and in all of them this type of opting out is heavily used. In fact, a 2006 study at the Johns Hopkins School of Public Health found that between 1991 and 2004, the number of unvaccinated children in states with philosophical exemptions more than doubled.

Nonetheless, anti-vaccinationists have become more aggressive in fighting to maintain or gain the right in their state to reject a vaccine for personal reasons. Jini Patel Thompson says, "It is very difficult to stand strong and resolute against the ubiquitous pressure to vaccinate. It's like having to keep insisting the earth is round when authorities, your community, intellectuals, and the majority of scientists etc. all insist it's flat. As with all matters of health, each of us has to go with what our gut tells us is right, or the best possible option for us at that time."[56]

Opponents of philosophical exemptions, however, insist that these views are based on fear stoked by misinformation. They argue that vaccine refusers should not be allowed to make choices that affect the health and well-being of other residents and that supersede those of qualified medical professionals. Walter Orenstein, for example, argues that people requesting philosophical exemptions should have to be educated on the subject of vaccines before the exemption can be granted. He says, "I believe

> "It should be a parent's choice, this should be a free country."[54]
>
> — Nicole Matten, who blames a vaccination for her seven-year-old daughter's death.

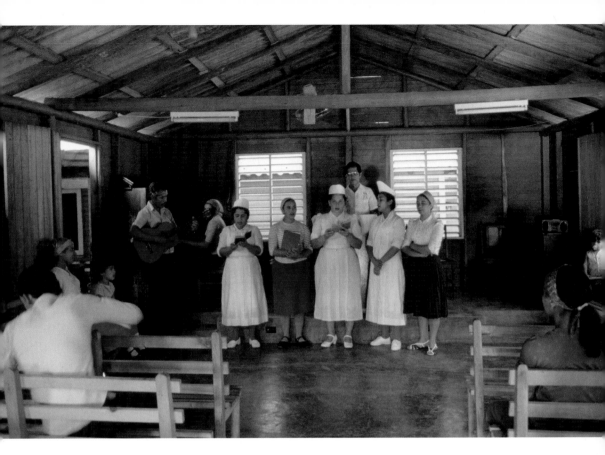

that a decision *not* to vaccinate is of equal gravitas to [the decision] *to* vaccinate. And there should be a procedure whereby people have to read information, understand information, and sign that they understand the risks they are putting that child through."[57]

Other vaccine proponents point out that people requesting such exemptions are not just putting themselves and their own children at risk but others as well. Therefore, these experts say, the issue is not one of personal freedom but of personal responsibility. For example, Amy Pisani, executive director of a pro-vaccination organization called Every Child by Two, says, "The question at hand is whether individuals have the right to shirk the laws put in place to maintain the health of some of Vermont's most vulnerable citizens, infants and school children."[58]

Christian Scientists, who believe that prayer is the only cure for illness, attend a prayer meeting. In the 1960s members of the Christian Science faith lobbied New York legislators for a religious exemption from vaccinating their children.

Religious Freedom

As with personal freedom, Americans have always placed high value on religious freedom. In conflicts between religious freedom and public health, however, the courts have had mixed rulings on whether a person's faith outweighs public health concerns. Many, however, have been guided by a 1940s US Supreme Court ruling involving a member of the Jehovah's Witnesses religion who forced her children to preach with her at night in violation of state labor laws. In its decision, the court stressed that child labor laws were important for a child's health and well-being, suggesting that being out at night could make the child sick. As part of this discussion the court said, "The right to practice religion freely does not include liberty to expose the community or the child to communicable disease or the latter to ill health or death."[59] This part of the ruling was seized upon by those wanting to stop resistance to mandatory vaccination.

In 1966, however, New York State passed a bill that allowed children to skip vaccinations for religious reasons and still attend school. This was the result of intense lobbying by members of the Christian Science religion. Members of this faith believe that all illnesses, even ones caused by a contagious disease, are the result of a disorder of the mind, not the body, and that prayer is the only cure needed for any illness. However, because other court rulings had already established that all religious groups had to be treated equally, members of religions with other beliefs were soon able to gain religious exemptions as well. Consequently more states decided to allow the exemptions under the assumption that the Supreme Court would consider it unconstitutional if they did not, and today forty-eight states provide them.

> "The question at hand is whether individuals have the right to shirk the laws put in place to maintain the health of some of Vermont's most vulnerable citizens, infants and school children."[58]
>
> — Amy Pisani of the pro-vaccination organization Every Child by Two.

Reasons for Refusing

The reasons given for requesting a religious exemption vary because religious faiths differ on which vaccines should be rejected and why. For example, members of religions that teach that it is wrong to consume certain animals might reject vaccines made using parts of those animals. (Fetal calf serum, for example, is used in the production of many vaccines.) Other people believe that injecting anything made from any kind of life form into a person's body is wrong because of a biblical verse that reads, "Thou shalt not let thy cattle gender with a diverse kind: thou shalt not sow thy field with mingled seed: neither shall a garment mingled of linen [plant] and woolen [animal] come upon thee."[60] Similarly, people who oppose abortion, such as Catholics, might reject only live-virus vaccines that have been cultivated from fetal cell lines that began with tissue from an aborted fetus. There are also those who try to turn their belief that vaccines are toxic into a religious excuse. For example, an exemption request letter posted on the Internet begins, "A conflict arises because my religious convictions are predicated on the belief that all life is sacred. God's commandment 'Thou Shall Not Kill' applies to the practice of injection of carcinogenic substances that can kill."[61]

Some would say this reason is not the kind of excuse the creators of religious exemptions had in mind—but at least it might reflect the petitioner's true beliefs. In some cases, however, people lie about their religious beliefs in order to gain an exemption. In coming up with lies that gain exemptions, they often turn to the Internet, where anti-vaccinationists help one another figure out ways to get around state vaccination laws. For example, on one website aimed at mothers, a post began this way: "What religions don't vaccinate?" It went on to say that the poster's family was moving to Hawaii, and she was searching for ways to get a religious or medical exemption from vaccinations for her children. She asked, "Anyone know how to get around vaccinating my children."[62] In response, readers posted many suggestions as well as links to websites and standard exemption request letters.

Rather than lie, some parents avoid vaccination requirements by homeschooling their children. Kansas mother Jill Craven, for example, chooses to homeschool her children specifically so she will not have to lie to public officials. At a meeting of lawmakers discussing the addition of a philosophical exemption to Kansas law in 2012, Craven said that since her faith did not oppose immunizations, a "conscientious objection" exemption would allow her to send her children to public schools "without having to

"The right to practice religion freely does not include liberty to expose the community or the child to communicable disease or the latter to ill health or death."[59]

— US Supreme Court.

lie."[63] Without this exemption, she would continue to homeschool rather than pretend to have a religious belief she did not have.

Toughening Requirements

Many states have considered demanding proof from people who claim their religious beliefs preclude vaccination. In 2011 New Jersey legislators considered just such a law, requiring those seeking a religious exemption to prove that their children were really being raised under the tenets of that religion by providing a baptismal certificate or other evidence of church membership or attendance. Ultimately, the state decided that a written statement from parents explaining how the vaccine violates their beliefs would be sufficient, but many people believe that even this is a violation of a person's right to privacy in regard to religious beliefs.

Others say it is wrong to make judgments regarding which belief should entitle someone to an exemption. This was the complaint of Gary McCormick after he and four others were fired in 2009 from their jobs at the Children's Hospital of Philadelphia for refusing a required flu shot. The hospital had mandated the vaccination as a condition of continuing employment because many of its patients are too sick or too young to be vaccinated, and exposure to the flu could kill them. However, they allowed exemptions for certain medical and religious beliefs, providing those exempted wore masks when near patients.

To determine who would be exempted, the hospital asked vaccine refusers to sign a waiver stating their reasons for refusing. These statements were then evaluated by a panel that also looked at each person's medical records to see whether the person had been vaccinated in the past. According to the hospital, both components of the application were used to determine sincerity of belief. The fired workers, who had all claimed religious exemptions, said it was not fair that they had been denied while others had not. McCormick says, "We're at a loss in terms of how does an institution make a determination of somebody's spiritual and religious beliefs and say, 'For you it's OK, but for you it's not OK.'"[64]

But Phil Plait, a blogger with *Discover* magazine, says, "This isn't a religious issue. It's a *safety* issue." By way of explanation,

Pandemic Threats

Under the Public Readiness and Emergency Preparedness Act (PREP), enacted by the Bush Administration in 2006, the US government has the power to force vaccination during a national emergency. Under this law, certain individual rights are set aside so that anyone who refuses to be vaccinated can be jailed without trial and without legal counsel as a "threat to national security." The law was enacted in response to concerns that terrorists might use biological weapons to create a pandemic that would weaken the United States. However, experts say that a pandemic is more likely to occur as the result of two subtypes of a virus encountering one another in the same host. If a human influenza A virus, for example, were to infect a pig (as has happened, beginning in 1998) and that pig were to also be infected by an avian influenza A virus, then a new virus with elements of both the human and the avian virus could be created by the mixing of the viruses. The resulting new virus would then be capable of infecting humans, who would not have any natural immunity to it because their bodies would never have encountered it before.

he compares vaccine refusal with another hospital requirement to keep people safe from disease: "Imagine someone at a hospital claiming their religion says they can't wash their hands! If I saw a hospital employee leave the bathroom without washing, I'd file a complaint instantly. I have no qualms with the hospital making vaccinations a mandatory requirement."[65]

Litigating Rights

In this case, the workers are settling their grievance with the hospital out of court. In other cases, vaccine refusers have engaged in lawsuits to fight for rights they feel have been taken away by vaccination policies. Many of these lawsuits relate to whether a person has a right to work in a certain place or attend a certain school without meeting the vaccine requirements of the workplace or school.

In a 2009 case Jennifer Workman of West Virginia sued the board of education because her school district would not allow her seven-year-old daughter to attend public school unless the girl received vaccinations against the common childhood diseases. In requiring this, the school district was following state law. However, state law also allows religious and medical exemptions, and Workman thought she met the criteria for both. First, she was a member of the Baptist Church, which teaches that a parent should not subject a child to medical harm. Second, Workman had gotten a certificate from a child psychiatrist saying that the shot would cause emotional and perhaps developmental harm to the girl. This was because Workman's older daughter had developed autism shortly after receiving an earlier vaccination.

Workman argued that her religious rights were being violated, but the district court dismissed her case, saying she had no grounds to sue. Workman continued pressing her case, however, and eventually it reached the US Supreme Court. But the court refused to hear the case, letting stand a ruling of a lower court that declared, "Workman does not explain how the statute at issue [the mandatory vaccination law] is facially discriminatory; indeed, her complaint is not that it targets a particular religious belief but that it provides no exception from general coverage for hers."[66]

In responding to the Supreme Court's decision to let this stand, John W. Whitehead of the Rutherford Institute, a group that supported Workman in her lawsuit, said, "It is unfortunate that the Supreme Court sidestepped this important constitutional issue. If the state is going to allow some exemptions from the vaccination requirement—which it should do—then a proper regard for religious freedom compels it to recognize religious exemptions as well."[67]

Homeschooling

Unable to gain an exemption, Workman turned to homeschooling, just as Craven did. Many vaccine refusers go that route, as do people who believe traditional schools are bad for their children in other ways. According to the National Home Education Research Institute, in 2010 there were about 2.04 million home-educated students in the United States, and this number is growing. Consequently lawmakers are now questioning whether homeschooled children should continue to be exempt from mandatory vaccination laws, especially since they are often involved in outbreaks. In 2008, for example, during one measles outbreak in Chicago, Illinois, twenty-five of the thirty cases involved unvaccinated homeschooled children. During another outbreak in Washington that same year, eleven of nineteen cases involved such children.

Ethicist Arthur Caplan of the University of Pennsylvania argues that vaccination is a public health issue and as such should be required for all children regardless of the type of school they

A homeschooling mother in Maine works with her children. Many parents who object to vaccinations for their children have turned to homeschooling to avoid laws that require vaccinations before students can start school.

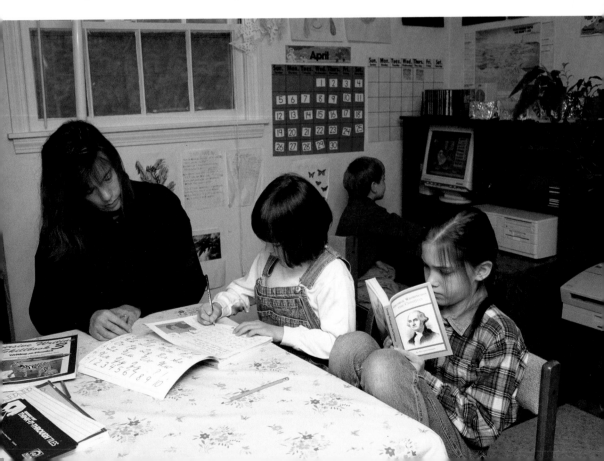

attend. Homeschooling parents counter that since their children do not spend time with other children in a classroom, their risk of spreading disease to others is minimal. But experts point out that people of all ages can be affected by contagious children who are not yet showing signs that they are carrying a dangerous disease. As Caplan notes, "Unvaccinated children pose not only a risk to themselves, but to their families, other children they come in contact with and especially older people they might visit or encounter in a movie theater or mall."[68]

Debate in Kansas

This issue of an unvaccinated person spreading risk into a community was at the forefront of public debates in Kansas in 2012 over adding a philosophical exemption to state vaccination laws. People opposed to allowing a new way to opt out of shots argued that preventing vaccination avoidance would be for the good of all. For example, David A. Smith, a Kansas public health official, said, "There are things that as a society we do because they're in the interest of the entire society and there are times when the collective well-being trumps our individual rights and it has to in order for our society to function well."[69]

"The state is essentially saying that those individuals harmed or killed by vaccines are necessary for the greater good. I find this abhorrent and offensive."[70]

— Pharmacist Erik Leon.

Others, however, argued that in taking this position, health officials like Smith were asking individuals to violate their principles and risk their health, and possibly their lives, for a cause they do not believe in. For example, Kansas pharmacist and parent Erik Leon said, "The state is essentially saying that those individuals harmed or killed by vaccines are necessary for the greater good. I find this abhorrent and offensive."[70] Kansas lawmakers ultimately decided not to support the exemption.

Risks and Consequences

The recent increase in outbreaks of vaccine-preventable diseases has led to media reports about the risks and consequences associated with such diseases. Some believe that this sort of attention, along with other efforts to inform the public, can influence opin-

Losing Parental Rights over a Vaccine

In 2012 a Pennsylvania newborn was taken away from her parents because of a refused hepatitis B vaccination. The parents, Scott and Jodi Ferris, had planned on a home birth but called for an ambulance after Jodi went into labor prematurely. At the Hershey Medical Center, nurses wanted to give the baby a hepatitis B shot, routinely given to infants to protect them in case their mothers have passed the virus to them prior to birth. Jodi said she would only agree to this after they tested to see whether she or the baby was positive for the virus because negative tests would mean the baby did not need the vaccine. Instead of conducting the test the hospital took custody of the baby on the grounds that the little girl's health was in danger, and a social worker officially approved the shot. Jody was then discharged from the hospital and only allowed to see her daughter every three hours in order to nurse the newborn. Although the Ferrises later had their rights reinstated, they are suing the hospital for violating these rights.

ions on vaccination. According to the Bloomberg news organization in 2012, roughly 85 percent of parents who had refused to vaccinate their children decided to allow vaccination after attending group information sessions at the Vaccine Education Center at Children's Hospital of Philadelphia. Consequently a *Bloomberg View* editorial argues that states should require anyone requesting a vaccination exemption to attend similar education sessions before the exemption can be granted. Otherwise, the editorial asserts, "One way or another, parents who eschew vaccination are going to learn they've made a mistake. Smallpox, a great affliction in early America, was almost defeated with a vaccine in the 1800s. When the disease was forgotten and immunization neglected, in the mid-1800s, it again became a mighty killer and had to be fought all over again. It would be better not to relive that experience with [other vaccine-preventable diseases]."[71]

But anti-vaccinationists typically believe that rejection of vaccines is prudent and that it is the other side that needs more information. To the most passionate of the deniers, editorials such as the one in *Bloomberg View* are an attempt to use scare tactics to manipulate behavior. For example, Ian Sinclair, a prominent Australian anti-vaccinationist until his death from a chronic illness in 2007, wrote in his 1992 book *Vaccination: The Hidden Facts*:

> When it comes to vaccination, the public are warned of severe epidemics, deaths and disabilities, killer diseases, maimed victims etc should . . . vaccination be stopped. In one newspaper article, the heading was titled "Immunize or Die!—Doc Warns." Is it any wonder that most people line up for their vaccinations? Obviously most people are not in a position to judge for themselves the validity of such claims and therefore are easily persuaded into accepting vaccinations, much to the delight of the vaccine industry. What the majority of the public do not realize, is that in most cases, if not all, such scare tactics are completely unfounded.[72]

Sinclair distrusted all claims that denying vaccines would have dire consequences. He believed that vaccination only exists to bring money to pharmaceutical companies and power and prestige to health experts. He never accepted the idea that vaccines might be necessary, no matter what arguments were presented to him. Many of today's anti-vaccinationists share this resolve, frustrating health experts who worry that a spread of vaccine denial will be accompanied by a spread of vaccine-preventable diseases that will threaten millions of individuals.

Facts

- In Australia parents can be cut off from child care benefit payments if their children have not had all of their mandated vaccines at the appropriate times.

- Between 2000 and 2010, immunization rates among health care providers at the Children's Hospital of Philadelphia rose from 35 percent to 99.9 percent, as a mandate for vaccination was implemented among workers.

- Some states allow exemptions to vaccination for those who can prove they are already naturally immune to the disease, which can be shown by measuring the level of antibodies to the disease in a person's blood.

- During the 2011–12 school year, Mississippi—the only US state that does not allow exemptions for religious or philosophical reasons—had a statewide total of only 16 kindergarten vaccine exemptions (for medical reasons), which according to the CDC represents essentially a 100 percent vaccination rate.

- According to the CDC, Washington state, which recognizes exemptions for medical, religious, and philosophical reasons, had the highest vaccine exemption rate of all 50 states, 6.2 percent.

- Between the 2009–10 school year and the 2011–12 school year, Arkansas had the largest increase in vaccine exemptions among kindergarteners, 650 percent, whereas Nebraska had the biggest decline, a more than 50 percent drop in vaccine exemptions.

Source Notes

Introduction: A Matter of Health?

1. Quoted in Sue Thomas, "After Losing Their Baby to Whooping Cough, Michigan Couple Channels Grief into Effort to Save Lives," Mlive.com, July 24, 2012. www.mlive.com.

2. Paula Simons, "Whooping Cough Outbreak: Pertussis and the Death-Rattle of Reason," *Edmonton (AB) Journal*, July 25, 2012. http://blogs.edmontonjournal.com.

3. Barbara Loe Fisher, "Vaccine Freedom of Choice," October 16, 2008. www.nvic.org.

Chapter One: What Are the Origins of the Modern Vaccination Controversy?

4. Quoted in Shari Roan, "Swine Flu 'Debacle' of 1976 Is Recalled," *Los Angeles Times*, April 27, 2009. http://articles.latimes.com.

5. Bob Guinter, "My Thoughts: Proof Is Powerful That Shots Save Lives," *Commercial Appeal*, March 25, 2012. www.commercialappeal.com.

6. Quoted in Roan, "Swine Flu 'Debacle' of 1976 Is Recalled."

7. Quoted in Lewis Mehl-Madrona, "Vaccines: The DPT Vaccine," Healing Center Online. www.healing-arts.org.

8. Harold Stearley, "The Tainted History of the DPT Vaccine," Commentary, *Albion Monitor*, April 18, 1997. www.monitor.net.

9. Quoted in Bob Greene, "Child Dies Despite Best of Intentions," *Chicago Tribune*, July 21, 1985. http://articles.chicagotribune.com.

10. Judy Converse, "Wakefield Has Company," Vaccination News, 2012. www.vaccinationnews.com.

11. Catherine J. Frompovich, "Murdoch's Vaccine World," Vactruth.com, July 22, 2011. http://vactruth.com.

12. Brian Deer. http://briandeer.com.

Chapter Two: Are Vaccines Safe?

13. Quoted in Jonathan D. Rockoff, "Scrutinized in Japan, Pfizer's Prevnar Vaccine Is Used Widely in U.S.," *Health Blog, Wall Street Journal*, March 7, 2011. http://blogs.wsj.com.

14. Elizabeth Birt Center for Autism Law and Advocacy (EBCALA), "Inadequate Vaccine Safety Research and Conflicts of Interest." www.ebcala.org.

15. Quoted in Stephanie Cave, *What Your Doctor May Not Tell You About Children's Vaccinations*. New York: Wellness Central, 2010, p. 25.

16. CDC, "Some Common Misconceptions About Vaccination," February 18, 2011. www.cdc.gov.

17. CDC, "Some Common Misconceptions About Vaccination."

18. NNII, "Cause or Coincidence," August 28, 2006. www.immunization info.org.

19. Paul A. Offit, *Deadly Choices: How the Anti-vaccine Movement Threatens Us All*. New York: Basic Books, 2011, p. 28.

20. Paul Gallagher, "Judy Wilyman's Vaccine Woo," *Losing in the Lucky Country* (blog), March 12, 2012. http://luckylosing.com.

21. Robert W. Sears, "Should You Insist on a Mercury-Free Flu Shot for Your Child?," MetroKids, January 2010. www.metrokids.com.

22. CDC, "Possible Side-Effects from Vaccines." www.cdc.gov.

23. Robert W. Sears, *The Vaccine Book*. New York: Little, Brown, 2011, p. 277.

24. Vaccine Education Center, Children's Hospital of Philadelphia, "Aluminum in Vaccines," Spring 2009. www.chop.edu.

25. Quoted in Lewis Mehl-Madrona, "How Could Children's Vaccines Cause Damage?," Healing Center Online, 2009. www.healing-arts.org.

Chapter Three: Should the HPV Vaccination Be Required?

26. Quoted in Dan Eggen, "Rick Perry Backs Away from HPV Vaccine Decision During Presidential Run," *Washington Post*, August 16, 2011. www.washingtonpost.com.

27. CDC, "HPV Vaccination Information for Young Women," July 17, 2012. www.cdc.gov.

28. Meghan O'Rourke, "Does the HPV Vaccine Promote Promiscuity?," *Slate*, September 27, 2007. www.slate.com.

29. Nancy Gibbs, "Defusing the War over the 'Promiscuity' Vaccine," *Time*, June 21, 2006. www.time.com.

30. Gibbs, "Defusing the War over the 'Promiscuity' Vaccine."

31. Shobha S. Krishnan, "Does the HPV Vaccine Promote Teen Promiscuity?," She Knows, September 23, 2008. www.sheknows.com.

32. Quoted in Adrian G. Uribarri, "Proposal to Require HPV Vaccination Stirs Concerns," *Los Angeles Times*, February 12, 2007. http://articles.la times.com.

33. Quoted in Uribarri, "Proposal to Require HPV Vaccination Stirs Concerns."

34. Quoted in Gibbs, "Defusing the War over the 'Promiscuity' Vaccine."

35. Quoted in Gibbs, "Defusing the War over the 'Promiscuity' Vaccine."

36. O'Rourke, "Does the HPV Vaccine Promote Promiscuity?"

37. Krishnan, "Does the HPV Vaccine Promote Teen Promiscuity?"

38. Quoted in American Academy of Neurology, "Researchers: Guillain-Barré Syndrome After HPV Vaccine Needs Monitoring," press release, February 13, 2009. www.aan.com.

39. Sears, *The Vaccine Book*, p. 160.

40. Sears, *The Vaccine Book*, p. 161.

Chapter Four: What Are the Consequences of Refusing Vaccinations?

41. Quoted in Allie Morris, "Ind. Measles Outbreak, Linked to Super Bowl, Raises Vaccination Concerns," Rundown, *PBS Newshour*, February 20, 2012. www.pbs.org.

42. Cave, *What Your Doctor May Not Tell You About Children's Vaccinations*, p. 20.

43. Quoted in Cave, *What Your Doctor May Not Tell You About Children's Vaccinations*, p. 20.

44. Vaccination Risk Awareness Network (VRAN), "'Herd Immunity': The Misplaced Driver of Universal Vaccination." http://vran.org.

45. Quoted in Vaccination Risk Awareness Network (VRAN), "Herd Immunity."

46. Jini Patel Thompson, "Should I Vaccinate My Child?," HealingWell.com. www.healingwell.com.

47. Vaccine Education Center, Children's Hospital of Philadelphia, "Hot Topics: Natural Infection vs. Immunization." www.chop.edu.

48. Quoted in Shirley S. Wang, "More Doctors 'Fire' Vaccine Refusers," *Wall Street Journal*, February 13, 2012. http://online.wsj.com.

49. Amanda Marcotte, "Measles Outbreak Traced to Super Bowl Anti-Vaccination Fanatics," XXfactor, *Slate*, February 24, 2012. www.slate.com.

50. Quoted in Morris, "Ind. Measles Outbreak."

51. Jennifer G. Cooke and Farhar Tahir, *Polio in Nigeria: The Race to Eradication*, CSIS Global Health Policy Center report, February 2012, p. 10. http://csis.org.

52. Quoted in Offit, *Deadly Choices*, pp. xvii–xviii.

53. Quoted in Dara Mohammadi, "The Final Push for Polio Eradication," *Lancet*, vol. 380, no. 9840, August 4, 2012. www.thelancet.com.

Chapter Five: Does Mandating Vaccines Violate People's Rights?

54. Quoted in Lara Salahi, "Vermont Debates Vaccines: Should Parents Be Able to Opt Out?," *ABC World News*, April 25, 2012. http://abcnews .go.com.

55. Quoted in Salahi, "Vermont Debates Vaccines."

56. Thompson, "Should I Vaccinate My Child?"

57. Quoted in Offit, *Deadly Choices*, p. 196.

58. Quoted in Salahi, "Vermont Debates Vaccines."

59. Quoted in Offit, *Deadly Choices*, p. 140.

60. Lev. 19:19.

61. Jen, "What Religions Don't Vaccinate?," Mothering. www.mothering .com.

62. Jen, "What Religions Don't Vaccinate?"

63. Quoted in Brad Cooper and Dawn Bormann, "Kansans Debate Vaccine Exemption," *Kansas City (MO) Star*, January 19, 2012. www.kansascity .com.

64. Quoted in Byron Scott, "Fired CHOP Couple: Religion Kept Them from Getting Vaccinated," NBC10 Philadelphia, December 7, 2009. www .nbcphiladelphia.com.

65. Phil Plait, "Hospital Workers Fired for Refusing Vaccinations," *Bad Astronomy* (blog), *Discover Magazine*, December 5, 2009. http://blogs.dis covermagazine.com.

66. Quoted in Jessica M. Karmasek, "U.S. Supreme Court Won't Hear W.Va. Vaccination Case," *West Virginia Record*, November 15, 2011. www.wv record.com.

67. Quoted in Karmasek, "U.S. Supreme Court Won't Hear W.Va. Vaccination Case."

68. Quoted in Chris Joyner, "Parents Home-School to Avoid Vaccinating Their Kids," *USA Today*, December 22, 2008. www.usatoday.com.

69. Quoted in Cooper and Dawn Bormann, "Kansans Debate Vaccine Exemption."

70. Quoted in Cooper and Bormann, "Kansans Debate Vaccine Exemption."

71. *Bloomberg View*, "Make It Hard for Parents to Deny Their Kids Vaccines," August 9, 2012. www.bloomberg.com.

72. Ian Sinclair, *Vaccination: The Hidden Facts*. Published by author, 1992. www.soilandhealth.org.

Related Organizations and Websites

American Academy of Family Physicians (AAFP)

11400 Tomahawk Creek Pkwy.
Leawood, KS 66211
phone: (800) 274-2237
e-mail: fp@aafp.org
website: www.aafp.org

One of the largest national medical organizations, the AAFP provides information on many aspects of young people's health, including vaccinations. The website also allows searches for AAFP "News Now" articles that report on vaccination issues and related current events.

American Academy of Pediatrics (AAP)

141 Northwest Point Blvd.
Elk Grove Village, IL 60007
phone: (800) 433-9016
website: www.aap.org

An organization of pediatricians committed to optimizing the physical and mental health of young people, the AAP provides information on many aspects of child, teen, and young adult health. To this end, its website offers guidelines on vaccinations and links to vaccination-related articles and reports.

American Medical Association

515 N. State St.
Chicago, IL 60654
phone: (800) 621-8335
website: www.ama-assn.org

This organization has promoted public health for over 160 years, and its website provides information on a variety of health issues, including vaccinations. The association also publishes one of the premier medical journals in the world, the *Journal of the American Medical Association (JAMA)*.

Centers for Disease Control and Prevention (CDC)

1600 Clifton Rd.
Atlanta, GA 30333
phone: (800) 232-4636; hotline: (800) 232-2522
e-mail: cdcinfo@cdc.gov
website: www.cdc.gov

The CDC, which operates under the US Department of Health and Human Services, is one of the premier public health organizations in the United States. Its website provides a wealth of information on all aspects of health, including the subject of vaccinations.

Every Child by Two

1233 20th St. NW, Suite 403
Washington, DC 20036
phone: (202) 783-7034
e-mail: info@ecbt.org
website: www.ecbt.org

This organization promotes the idea that it is critical for children to get their vaccinations by the age of two and provides information on vaccinations and diseases that can be prevented by vaccinations.

Global Vaccine Awareness League

phone: (866) 888-2901
website: www.gval.com

Established by a woman who believes her child was killed by a DPT shot, this anti-vaccination website provides support for parents who want to refuse vaccinations. Its website also includes information about state exemptions related to vaccinations.

Immunization Action Coalition

1573 Selby Ave., Suite 234
St. Paul, MN 55104
phone: (651) 647-9009
e-mail: admin@immunize.org
website: www.immunize.org

This group works to increase immunization rates through education. To this end, its website has a great deal of information on vaccines, as well as downloadable handouts related to diseases and vaccines.

Infectious Diseases Society of America (IDSA)

1300 Wilson Blvd., Suite 300
Arlington, VA 22209
phone: (703) 299-0200
website: www.idsociety.org

The IDSA is a group for physicians and other professionals involved in combating infectious diseases. However, it also promotes public health and prevention efforts as they relate to infectious diseases, and its website provides news reports and other information related to vaccinations.

Institute for Vaccine Safety

Johns Hopkins Bloomberg School of Public Health
615 N. Wolfe St., Room W5041
Baltimore, MD 21205
e-mail: info@vaccinesafety.edu
website: www.vaccinesafety.edu

Established in 1997, this organization independently assesses vaccines to help guide policy on vaccine safety and to support public education efforts. Its website provides current information on contagious diseases, vaccines, and vaccine safety.

National Childhood Vaccine Injury Compensation Program

Parklawn Bldg., Room 11C-26
5600 Fishers Ln.
Rockville, MD 20857
phone: (800) 338-2382
website: www.hrsa.gov

Created as a result of the National Childhood Injury Act of 1986 in order to ensure that US pharmaceutical companies would continue to manufacture vaccines, this government program resolves vaccine injury claims using a no-fault system that prevents lawsuits. The program's website provides information on how to file a claim regarding suspected injury from a vaccine and offers data and statistics related to vaccines.

National Institutes of Health (NIH)

9000 Rockville Pike
Bethesda, MD 20892
phone: (301) 496-4000
e-mail: nihinfo@od.nih.gov
website: www.nih.gov

An agency of the US Department of Health and Human Services, the NIH is responsible for research into issues related to public health, and this includes vaccine-related studies. Its website therefore provides a great deal of information related to vaccines, including fact sheets and statistics related to clinical trials.

National Network for Immunization Information (NNII)

website: www.immunizationinfo.org

An affiliation of several medical associations that include the Infectious Disease Society of America, the American Medical Association, and the American Academy of Pediatrics, this group provides health professionals, policy makers, and the public with current scientific information related to immunization.

National Vaccine Information Center (NVIC)
407 Church St., Suite H
Vienna, VA 22180
phone: (703) 938-0342
e-mail: contactnvic@gmail.com
website: www.nvic.org

Founded in 1982, this organization promotes vaccine safety and works to protect the right to informed consent in the public health system.

Think Twice Global Vaccine Institute
website: http://thinktwice.com

Established in 1996, this organization provides information and support for those who want to reject vaccinations, although it also seeks to help pro-vaccination parents make informed choices on individual vaccines.

US Food and Drug Administration (FDA)
10903 New Hampshire Ave.
Silver Spring, MD 20993
phone: (888) 463-6332
e-mail: webmail@oc.fda.gov
website: www.fda.gov

An agency of the US Department of Health and Human Services, the FDA is responsible for the regulation and supervision of products and procedures related to public health. This includes vaccines, so the agency's website provides information on vaccine safety and related issues.

Vaccination Liberation Network
website: www.vaclib.org

This anti-vaccination website provides anti-vaccine information and offers support to people wanting to refuse vaccines.

The Vaccine Times

website: www.vaccinetimes.com

This pro-vaccination website provides a wealth of scientific information, statistics, and news reports related not only to vaccinations but to disease outbreaks around the world.

World Health Organization (WHO)

Ave. Appia 20
1211 Geneva 27
Switzerland
phone: + 41 22 791 21 11
website: www.who.int/en

Established in 1948, the WHO is an international organization
that promotes health efforts around the world. It has been at
the forefront of efforts to eradicate contagious diseases like polio
worldwide through vaccination programs and the promotion of
better sanitary practices. Its website includes information about
vaccination programs and statistics related to disease outbreaks.

Additional Reading

Books

Stephanie Cave with Deborah Mitchell, *What Your Doctor May Not Tell You About Children's Vaccinations.* New York: Wellness Central, 2010.

Don S. Dizon and Michael L. Krychman, *Questions & Answers About Human Papilloma Virus (HPV).* Sudbury, MA: Jones and Bartlett, 2011.

Louise Kuo Habakus, Mary Holland, and Kim Mack Rosenberg, eds., *Vaccine Epidemic: How Corporate Greed, Biased Science, and Coercive Government Threaten Our Human Rights, Our Health, and Our Children.* New York: Skyhorse, 2012.

Mark A. Largent, *Vaccine: The Debate in Modern America.* Baltimore: Johns Hopkins University Press, 2012.

Neil Z. Miller, *Vaccine Safety Manual for Concerned Families and Health Practitioners.* 2nd ed. Santa Fe, NM: New Atlantean, 2011.

Seth Mnookin, *The Panic Virus: A True Story of Medicine, Science, and Fear.* New York: Simon & Schuster, 2011.

Paul A. Offit, *Deadly Choices: How the Anti-Vaccine Movement Threatens Us All.* New York: Basic Books, 2011.

Robert W. Sears, *The Vaccine Book.* New York: Little, Brown, 2011.

Internet Sources

CDC, "Frequently Asked Questions About HPV Vaccine Safety." www.cdc.gov/vaccinesafety/Vaccines/HPV/hpv_faqs.html.

CDC, "Frequently Asked Questions About Vaccine Safety." www.cdc.gov/vaccinesafety/Vaccines/Common_questions.html.

Immunization Action Coalition, "Vaccine Concerns: Religious and Ethical Concerns Resources." www.immunize.org/concerns/religious.asp.

Albert D.M.E. Osterhaus, *Pandemics: Is Hoping for the Best Enough?* EMBO (European Molecular Biology Organization) Reports, 2010. www.nature.com/embor/journal/v11/n3/full/embor201022.html.

Imm Younity, "Vaccine Q & A: Truthful Information About Vaccines," Connaught Technology Corp. www.vaccines.com/vaccine-questions-answers.cfm.

Index

Note: Boldface page numbers indicate illustrations.

Picture Credits

About the Author

Patricia D. Netzley is the author of over fifty books for teens and adults. She also teaches writing and is a member of both the Society of Children's Books Writers and Illustrators and the Romance Writers of America.

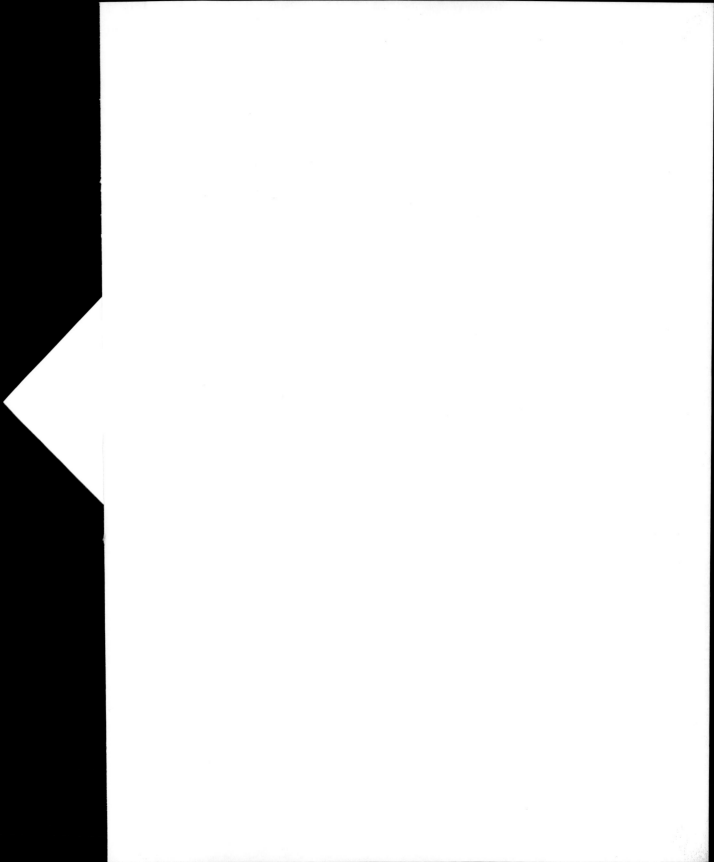

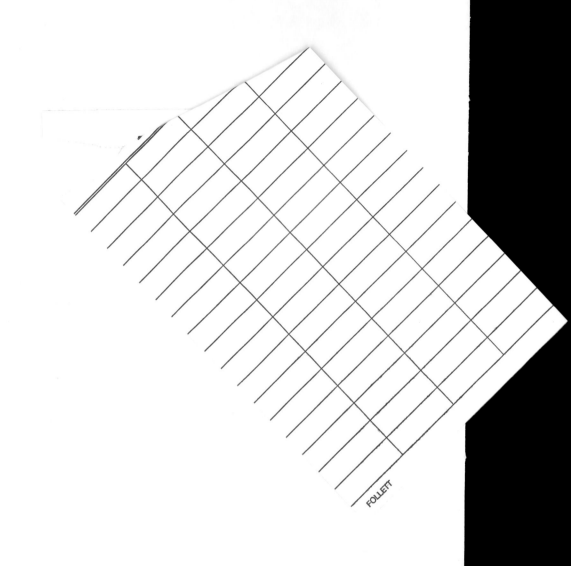